Successful Private Practice

A Guide to Effective Medical Practice Management

Susan Wynn-Williams MCSP
Susan Wynn-Williams qualified as a Chartered
Physiotherapist at the Queen Elizabeth, United
Birmingham Hospitals. She worked for eight years in
both the National Health Service and industry. After a
two year spell in public relations and advertising, she
returned to clinical work and purchased an established
private practice in London in 1974 with Maxine
Buchele which incorporated work for the Royal Ballet
School. In 1981, she sold the London practice and
formed Henley Physiotherapy Services, a group
practice in 1982. She is married with four grown-up
children.

Maxine Buchele BA (Hons) MCSP
Maxine Buchele qualified as a Chartered
Physiotherapist at Guy's Hospital, London. She
worked in the National Health Service for five years
and then gained both clinical and managerial
experience in the USA. On her return to the UK she
became superintendent physiotherapist of two London
hospitals. In 1973 she started a physiotherapy
employment agency and in 1974 joined in partnership
with Susan Wynn-Williams to buy a practice in
London. She gained a BA in 1983 and is currently
reading for a law degree.

Successful Private Practice

A Guide to Effective Medical
Practice Management

Maxine Buchele

Susan Wynn-Williams

Foreword by
John C. H. Strachan FRCS
Consultant Orthopaedic Surgeon,
Charing Cross Hospital, London;
The Royal Ballet Company;
The London Festival Ballet.

CHURCHILL LIVINGSTONE
EDINBURGH LONDON MELBOURNE AND NEW YORK 1987

CHURCHILL LIVINGSTONE
Medical Division of Longman Group UK Limited

Distributed in the United States of America by
Churchill Livingstone Inc., 1560 Broadway, New
York, N.Y. 10036, and by associated companies,
branches and representatives throughout the world.

First published 1987

ISBN 0 443 03456 7

British Library Cataloguing in Publication Data
Buchele, Maxine
    Successful private practice.
    1. Medicine——Practice
    I. Title   II. Wynn-Williams, Susan
    610'.68   R729.5G4

Library of Congress Cataloging in Publication Data
Buchele, Maxine.
    Successful private practice.
    Bibliography: p.
    Includes index.
    1. Medicine——Practice. 2. Medicine——Practice——
Great Britain.—I. Wynn-Williams, Susan. II. Title.
[DNLM: 1. Practice Management, Medical. 2. Private
Practice. W 89 B919s]
R728.B8 1986   610'.68   86–9547

Printed and bound in Great Britain by
William Clowes Limited, Beccles and London

Foreword

It gives me great pleasure to write the Foreword to this excellent book. The authors have gone into great detail to cover all aspects of private practice and it is a book that should be read carefully by anyone who is about to venture forth into an area in which one normally gets very little advice, and where it is possible to make quite serious mistakes both professionally and financially.

Careful perusal of this book should allow the reader to avoid nearly all those mistakes.

I was honoured to have been asked to write these few words, having studied this work carefully and noting the logical and sensible approach of the two authors who have tackled the problem in an extremely professional way.

J.C.H.S.

Preface

This book has been written for the medical and health care professions. In the years of being in private practice, many of our colleagues came to us for advice. Having established a successful private practice, we felt the business and management experience we gained, might prove helpful for those wishing to enter private practice for themselves.

We have tried to provide information which may also be useful for practitioners who already have established practices, but who may wish to expand and develop them in the future.

Although it is clear the book has been written from experience gained in the United Kingdom, the problems associated with both the business and clinical aspects of private practice are common to many other countries who have a strong tradition of private medical care, and we have included an Appendix for sources of information in certain countries.

We have tried to give practical solutions to common problems, such as credit control, after hours telephone calls and hiring personnel. We hope these solutions will help practitioners improve their working arrangements and assist decision-making.

We have emphasised the legal aspects of medical practice because of the increasing importance which legal matters have assumed in the practice of medicine and health care. Topics have been chosen and discussed to increase the practitioner's awareness of both the potential legal problems of conducting a medical practice and the need for continual competent advice.

In order to avoid confusion and the continual use of him or her we refer throughout the book to the patient as 'him' and the practitioner as 'you'. We hope you will like reading the book and find it a useful reference, and we hope it will help you achieve a practice where you will get enjoyment and the satisfaction which follows with success.

Henley-on-Thames, 1987   M.B
                                                                          S.W.-W.

Acknowledgements

In the preparation of this book we are grateful to the following people for their unstinting advice, interest and help:

Dr Ian Simpson from The Medical Defence Union, Dr Eric Blackadder, the Group Medical Adviser of BUPA and the legal department of American Health Care Ltd, for their advice and helpful criticism on the legal chapter of the book. Lord Denning for his kind permission to use an extract from one of his speeches. Heather Gordon of Midgley Snelling & Co., Chartered Accountants who has given invaluable advice for the accounting and financial material of the text. Mrs Penelope Robinson, Professional Adviser to the Chartered Society of Physiotherapy who has given us so much encouragement. Friends who are members of The Organisation of Chartered Physiotherapists in Private Practice. The British United Provident Association, American Health Care Ltd, Mrs M John, Mrs A McLauglin and Henley Physiotherapy Services for their kind permission to reproduce their photographs; Richard Cooksey who despite the weather, still managed to take good photographs, and Michael Linguane who processed them. Miss Lois Dyer, Remedial Adviser to the Department of Health and Social Security for her initial interest and introduction to our publishers.

In addition, we would like to thank all the overseas professional organisations who have helped in the compilation of the Appendix. We are indebted to the staff of Henley Public Library for their interest and professional help.

Last, but certainly not least, we would like to thank Annette Maiden and Julia Botteley who have kindly read the text, David Wynn-Williams who courageously undertook the photocopying, and finally, we wish to record our grateful thanks and appreciation to our secretaries, especially, Mrs Doreen Woodward who accepted the burden of typing the numerous drafts of this book from indecipherable copy.

M.B
S.W.-W.

Contents

1 WHAT IS PRIVATE PRACTICE?   1

A change in direction   2
Experience   3
Scope of practice   4
The time factor   4
Health   5
Stress   6
Income   7

Approaching the private sector   8

Where to practise?   9
A practice in your home town   9
Running a practice from home   9
Practising in premises   10
Domiciliary practice   11

The ways to practise   12
Single-handed practice   12
Partnership   13
Association or group practice   14
A limited company   14
Entering private practice on a part-time basis   14
As an assistant or locum   15

The advantages of private practice   15

2 STARTING IN PRIVATE PRACTICE   17

Choosing where   17
The community's need for a practitioner   17
Personal needs   18
Local medical facilities   19

Acquiring premises   20
The estate agent   20

The size and layout of the practice   21
Estimates and quotations   22
Time scale/factor   22

Planning permission and local authorities   23
Licences   24
Fire precautions   24

The property   24
Freehold property   25
Leasehold property   26
Renting property   26

Purchasing an existing practice   27
Why is the practice for sale?   27
What is for sale?   28
Scrutinising the practice finances   28
Evaluating the assets   28
Negotiating the price   31
Paying for the practice   32
The advantages of buying   32

Professional advisers   32
When to look for an accountant   33
The accountant   33
The solicitor   33
Where to look for an accountant and a solicitor   34
Fees   34
Insurance broker   34
The bank manager   35

3 FINANCIAL PLANNING AND MANAGEMENT   37

Running a business   37

Planning   37
The short-term plan   38
The long-term plan   38

Establishing costs   39
Setting up costs   39
Running costs   40
Hidden costs   40
Personal needs   41
Costing your fees   41

Budgeting and forecasting   42
A profit and loss account   44

Budgeting 44
Cash flow 44
The balance sheet 46
Forecasting 46

Sources of finance 50
Savings 50
Approaching the bank 50
Information for the bank manager and financial sources 51
Overdrafts 52
Bank loan 52
Partnership capital 52
Building societies 53
Government money and grants 53
Finance and leasing companies 53

Keeping accounts 54
Books of account 57
The day book 58
The cash book 58
The petty cash book and cash in the office 59
Cash deposits 59

Wages and salaries system 59
Pay As You Earn 60
National Insurance contributions 60
Contracts of employment 60

Taxation 61
The tax year 61
National Insurance contributions 61
Tax and marriage 61
Principal allowable business expenses 62
Stock valuation 63
Value Added Tax 63
Pensions and retirement 64
Investment advice 64
Reminder note 65

4 LEGAL IMPLICATIONS AND INSURANCE 66

Ethics
Rules of professional conduct 66

Medical practitioners and the law 67
The contract with the patient 67

Breach of contract   67
Negligence   68
Standard of care   69
Consent   69
Confidentiality   70
Vicarious liability   72
Chaperones   73

Professional conduct   74
Disciplinary procedures   74
Complaints   75

Keeping medical records   76
The appointment book   76

Advertising   76
Choosing a name or title for the practice   77
Professional door-plates   77
Announcing the opening of the practice   77
Sale of goods   78
Publicity and the media   78

Insurance   79
The contract with the insurance company   80
Surgery or practice insurance   80
Legal liability insurance   81
Car insurance   82
Personal accident insurance   82
Permanent health insurance   83
Private medical insurance   83
Drugs   83
Money   83
Mortgage minder   84
Life policies   84

Seeking legal advice   85
The courts   85
A partnership agreement   85
A limited company   87
The police   87
Conveyancing   87
Making a will   88
Legacies   88

5 OFFICE PLANNING AND MANAGEMENT   89

The office   89
Office furniture   89
The staff room   90
Prevention of theft   90
Fire extinguishers   91
Storage areas   91

Buying office furniture and equipment   92
Business office equipment   92

Communications   93
Telephone services   93
Answering machines   94
Answering service   94
Call divertors   95
Call systems   95
Car telephones and the cellular network   95
Yellow pages and other directories   96

Filing equipment and systems   96
Filing equipment   96
Filing systems and records   97
Computers   98

Printing and stationery   101
Letterheads   101
Professional cards   101
Appointment cards   102
Account forms   102
Medical record cards   103
An appointment book   103
An address book   103
Memo pads   104
Rubber stamps and labels   104
Office sundries   104
Mail and postage   104

Reference books   105

Transportation and the car   105
Buying the car   106
Running costs of the car   106

6 PRACTICE PLANNING AND MANAGEMENT   108

Decor   108
Colour schemes   108
Furnishings   109
Floor coverings   109
Walls and partitions   109
Corridors, passages and stairs   109
Windows, curtains and blinds   110
Lighting and mirrors   110
Heating and ventilation   110
The front door   110
A cleaner   111

The reception/waiting area   111

The receptionist/secretary   113
Telephone reception   114
Information notices   115

Consulting/treatment rooms   115
Linen and professional attire   116
Consultations   116

Buying medical equipment   119
Manufacturing and pharmaceutical companies   119
Where to buy equipment   120
The service engineer   120

Scheduling patients' appointments   120
Patient reminders   122

Accounts: method and collection   122
Fees   122
Rendering the account   123
Credit cards   123
Credit control   124

7 PERSONNEL AND HOSPITAL MANAGEMENT   128

Employing staff   128
Delegation   128
Recruitment and advertising   129
Job description, analysis and specification   129
Interviews   130
Personal qualities   131
Selection   132

Employing relatives   132
References   132

Contract of employment   133
Wages and salaries   133
Time off, holidays and sick leave   134
Safety at work   134

Practice policies   134
Personnel management and training   135
Keeping staff   136
Promotion   136
Discharging staff   137

Emergency staff   137
Locums   137
Agency staff   137

Consultancy   138
Hospital commissions   139

Hospital patient management   140
Private practice and national health care   140
Scheduling hospital visits   141
Admitting rights   141

Hospital employment   141
Job description   142
Interview   142
The contract   142
Informed consent   144
Recording hospital patients   145
Discharging patients from hospital   145
Follow-up appointments   146
Hospital patients' accounts   146

8 PRIVATE PRACTICE: PAST, PRESENT AND FUTURE 148

BIBLIOGRAPHY   153

RELEVANT ACTS OF PARLIAMENT   154

APPENDICES   155

Australia   157
Belgium   167

Canada   170
Denmark   178
Eire   180
Hong Kong   183
Japan   185
The Netherlands   186
New Zealand   189
Norway   191
South Africa   192
Sweden   194
Switzerland   195
United Kingdom   196
Northern Ireland   215
United States of America   216

INDEX   233

1

What is private practice?

The first of earthly blessings, independence.
Edward Gibbon 1737–1794

Private practice is an exciting and challenging venture. The freedom of choice for the individual is the essence of a democratic society. A large number of professional people work for themselves and this number is steadily increasing. In private practice the practitioner has complete and total independence, clinical responsibility for the patient, and overall charge of the administration and management of the business side of the practice.

Although a national health care system may offer a full range of treatment, many people choose to be treated privately. Private practice gives greater flexibility in terms of appointment or treatment times, and the continuity of individual attention by one practitioner from the initial consultation right through to the completion of treatment. National health care and private practice are not incompatible: they can, and do, exist side by side. The needs of the patient, therefore, can be met through a medical system which offers a highly desirable freedom of choice.

Many practitioners will continue to seek and find professional satisfaction and fulfilment within a national medical system, specialising, teaching or in research. Medicine in whatever form needs hard work, skill, energy, enthusiasm, dedication and patience. Private practice, however, demands particular qualities which are both personal and professional.

A private practitioner must have commitment and the ability to communicate well, and remain alert and versatile, enhancing and developing skills and techniques constantly so that a diverse range of conditions can be treated, from a foreign child with poliomyelitis to an elderly deaf patient with a chronic leg ulcer. It is well-treated patients who generate the goodwill which builds a practice.

The recent rapid growth and development of private health care has opened up many opportunities for those who have the

1

knowledge and skill to work for themselves. The practitioner may plan to start from scratch or develop an existing practice. If the opportunity arises to acquire a practice which offers suitable quiet and privacy for consulting or treatment rooms, then those who have already begun to think about private practice may wish to give serious consideration to buying one. All the aspects of working for oneself must be thought out very carefully before any conclusions can be reached.

Before making the final decision and considering personal circumstances, hopes and aspirations, a whole range of questions will come to mind. Will I like private practice? Is it suited to me as an individual? Where shall I practise? How shall I obtain patients? Have I the necessary business acumen? How do I set about acquiring premises? What about money, insurance, holidays? How will it affect me, my family and friends? Am I prepared for all the risks? Do I really know what it entails?

Whilst opportunities are constantly occurring in private practice, it is becoming increasingly competitive, and it would be an unwise person indeed who launched into private work without careful thought, reflection and planning.

Read on and decide for yourself whether a career in private practice is really what you want. Be optimistic, persevere, accept the consequences and enjoy the benefits.

A change in direction

The practitioner will probably be leaving a national health care system in which training and experience will have been obtained. Tax, insurance, pensions, holidays, study and sick leave are all arranged by the health care system and, very importantly, income is steady and assured. In private practice all these items are the responsibility of the practitioner and income may be very variable, especially in the early days.

Working in a hospital with other professionals offers the contact and companionship of colleagues. Except at a very senior level, little administrative work is required, but in private practice the administrative work must be done in addition to clinical work. Business management and patient care are almost indivisible. Private work can be lonely, with long irregular hours. Unless sufficient time is allowed, contact and communication with colleagues can be distant and this is a disadvantage. However, other health services are nearly always available in the neighbourhood.

Private practice is different; it alters your thinking and lifestyle. This change should be seen as a challenge and accepted, as the long-term benefits are very rewarding.

Experience

The formal training of the professional practitioner may vary from four to seven years, but once the qualification is obtained the real business of gaining experience and confidence begins. It is inadvisable to contemplate private practice without at least five years good general experience, plus training in any specialised areas which are of interest to the individual practitioner. It is only through constant contact with patients and their problems that the practitioner acquires the skill and expertise, composure and confidence necessary for professional private practice.

You will not succeed if your ability and skills are inadequate, or if you lack the maturity to deal with the problems private practice can bring. It can be difficult to change from clinical work in a hospital, where the support of colleagues is readily available, to an environment where you will be working on your own and will have to rely on your own skill and judgement. The physical detachment from the medical team can be lonely. Post-registration courses must be attended whenever possible, as familiarity with new techniques and ideas are essential for good practice.

It would be unreasonable to expect anybody to 'know it all' but a good clinical background is vital if complete patient care is to be given with competence and confidence. However, it is equally important to know your own limitations. Professional dignity and pride must never be allowed to stand in the way of good patient management. If you do not have the appropriate training and skill, you must refer a patient, whenever it is necessary, to another practitioner who has the knowledge and expertise. In addition to clinical skills, personal qualities are very important for successful practice. Original and creative thought, a well-developed sense of humour, enthusiasm, tremendous energy, a smiling friendly manner together with a soundly-based personal confidence, will go a long way to giving a patient confidence in *you*.

Administrative experience

Administrative ability is as important as appropriate clinical experience. It enables the practice to run smoothly and efficiently.

It is a skill that comes with management experience so that any problems are hidden from the patient and he feels completely at ease.

Scope of practice

Once you are fully trained and qualified you must confine yourself to the areas of practice in which you are trained. This at first may seem obvious, but in reality the definition of training is somewhat elusive.

Training in its formal sense may be seen as a body of knowledge, expertise and experience gained prior to qualification. The medical profession, as do other professions, changes and develops. New techniques, equipment and methods of treatment are constantly introduced, thus much knowledge and expertise is gained during a professional's lifetime. Training, therefore, will in a large part be outside the formal and academic, and new skills acquired in this way are quite acceptable provided they are practised properly and professionally. Do make sure, however, that what you intend to do is within the currently accepted scope of practice. If in doubt, ask your professional organisation.

A full assessment of the patient's history, signs and symptoms must be noted and recorded accurately as it is particularly important in private practice to keep well-written records. You may be the only qualified person to see the patient and any errors or omissions will, therefore, not be noticed by another practitioner. The legal implications of this are discussed in Chapter 4.

The time factor

The allocation and control of time deserves much consideration, both in your professional and personal life, if you are envisaging a successful practice and a reasonable lifestyle. Poor allocation of time will lead to fatigue, strain on the family and friends, and a generally disorganised and chaotic way of life. This is bad for a proper professional image, your personal well-being and the smooth running of the practice.

One of the main advantages for private practitioners is the additional time they have in which to listen and talk to the patient. He may be shy, nervous or sometimes very apprehensive, so the time given by a quiet, confident practitioner will put him at his ease. A busy, rushed practitioner who has failed to assign enough time, will only increase the patient's discomfort and worry, and he may therefore seek another source of treatment. The patient has chosen to consult you because he wants your advice and expertise. He does not wish to hear how difficult it was for you to park your car or that you have overslept! It is inevitable that you will be late for some appointments and the reason may be perfectly genuine. If you are delayed, apologise to the patient for keeping him waiting and then give him your whole and undivided attention.

Time must be spent on personal appearance. Clothes must be restrained, suitable, smart and, most important of all, clean and tidy. There has been a move over recent years towards a more informal style of clothing, but this casual trend has been very slow to reach the medical professions.

Well-groomed, tidy hair and clean manicured hands are essential, and close attention should be paid to personal hygiene.

You must allow sufficient time for family and friends, or problems and resentment will occur. Working hours will be unsocial. Time for emergencies must be found, as the patient has first priority, and unless you have made arrangements with another practitioner to cover your work, you will have to attend to the patient.

Certain times will have to be found for discussions with your professional advisers, for example, a solicitor or an accountant, who are essential for the efficient running of the business aspects of a successful private practice, and you will have to find time for plenty of communication with other medical colleagues.

The accounting systems, records and other paperwork will have to be kept and filed. Visits have to be made to the bank and the post office during working hours.

The control of time is a skill in itself, and it is important to master it, as the efficient use of time and your own self-discipline will be prime contributory factors to success.

Health

Working for yourself is not a soft option. Will your health stand the demands and self-discipline that private practice requires? If you are ill, there will be no earnings and patients will have to be cancelled unless you have made alternative arrangements. You will need great physical resilience and stamina. You must be fit, active and lively. Try and take some form of exercise at least once a week. Keep your weight at your personal average; eat sensibly and regularly. It is often impossible to take time for lunch during a busy practice day. Accept this fact, but eat a reasonable breakfast and a good meal in the evening. A healthy practitioner will enjoy private practice and this will show in the approach to patients and allow a high standard of care to be given.

Stress

This has been defined as 'a state of bodily or mental tension resulting from factors which tend to alter an existing equilibrium'. Going into private practice can be stressful as it demands a great deal in terms of time, energy, thinking and planning, and the ability to cope with an almost endless number of changes and problems which have not previously been encountered.

Self-employment may mean a drop in income, and therefore, initially, in your standard of living, until the practice starts to build up. You and your family must accept this from the outset. It may lead to a temporary feeling of insecurity and this can bring feelings of anxiety or strain. The long working hours may lead to tiredness, worry and fatigue, but as the practice succeeds you will be able to delegate some of the work and any serious long-term effects from too heavy a work-load will be avoided.

Contrary to the belief that stress is unavoidable, a certain degree of stress is necessary and many people seem to positively thrive on it. It depends on how you respond to its impact. You have to separate stress from distress. Know when you are at your optimum and full of energy, rather than overwhelmed by external pressures. The demands private practice make on you personally will have to be reviewed from time to time, so that you do not start thinking about them obsessively until eventually you lose the will to work.

However well motivated and enthusiastic you are, a life devoted to work is not healthy ultimately. Be positive about both your mental and physical health.

If you allow events to flow smoothly with a clear, decisive, realistic mind, everyday stresses will not tire you out. They will stimulate your drive, imagination and resourcefulness. Delays or obstacles you cannot control will be used as a time to think positively and concentrate on the progress you are making to reach your goals, instead of a time to become frustrated or discouraged and wonder what went wrong.

Certain groups of people can be identified as stress resistant. The characteristics which identify these people are:

discussion section

1. They seek out and welcome change, viewing it as a challenge with potential for growth and excitement.
2. They can identify a stressful situation and adapt to it quickly and do not waste energy and time fighting it; they defuse it instead of regarding the problem as alien and hostile.
3. They plan, set goals and solve their problems, feeling totally complete at the end of a task. There is no uncertainty but a sense of control and gratification.

There are several ways to learn stress management and reach a personal level of control:

1. Modify expectations and be flexible about plans and results.
2. Ask for feedback. Evaluate your performance from others. There will be those in a position to observe so find out if there are any criticisms.
3. Share and discuss problems. A problem shared is a problem halved.
4. Try and achieve a smooth-running practice. Conflicts can lead to a 'me and them' situation with unclear aims, whereas well-defined objectives will lead to closer relationships with colleagues.
5. Have rest and relaxation: try breathing exercises, postural movements and get a good night's sleep.
6. Make time for pleasureable events, such as seeing friends outside medicine, hobbies and family holidays.
7. Only do the type of physical exercise you enjoy; do not participate in sport because you feel you must: this will only bring about tension.

Severe fatigue leads to carelessness and errors. In medicine, these can be very serious. A proper balance must be struck between working hard and allowing time for leisure and relaxation.

You will then have control, confidence and authority; you will be able to think clearly and be prepared to have commitment to the patient. You must be strong minded enough to say 'no' to work without feeling guilty.

It might sound like the counsel of perfection and perhaps it is. It is certainly difficult to achieve, but both you and your practice will be more efficient, cheerful, pleasant and successful if you can.

Income

When you are considering private practice, you will have to decide what income you need from the practice. It will have to cover your monthly drawing requirements, however moderate, possibly a mortgage, all the overheads and running expenses, the car and staff. As a self-employed person you will not enjoy automatic sick pay, study leave or paid maternity leave. If there are no profits, you will not be able to draw money and will have to borrow from the bank or use other capital during this period. All aspects of the financial side of the business have important implications for you and your tax and financial position. These are described fully in Chapter 3.

If you are already running a home and looking after a family, you will have to weigh up the advantages and disadvantages of an anticipated income in private practice which, although a welcome addition to the family budget, could be at the expense of time spent with the family. Be realistic when you calculate how much money you need to sustain yourself—you cannot live on fresh air for too long!

APPROACHING THE PRIVATE SECTOR

Prior to commencing private practice, it is advisable to approach the professional organisation to which you belong. Most of the organisations have a member of staff dealing with initial enquiries and they may be able to send you some preliminary information. This may include national guidelines, rules of conduct and a general outline of what private practice entails. There may well be an organised network of regional representatives who can be contacted to answer questions or queries at a more local level.

It is advisable to contact and, where possible, meet other medical colleagues. The time to begin these contacts is several weeks before you start the practice. This may seem common sense, but often lack of communication leads to problems and difficulties. Although competition is healthy, obvious encroachment is very unprofessional and unwelcome and indirectly a poor reflection on the professions.

Make a list of all the health professionals who must be contacted and visited to spread the word about the practice, such as:

1. The administrator, consultants and staff at the local hospital, nursing home and health clinic to discuss medical practice generally in the area: find out if your services are required, the possibility of referrals and any special procedures which may be involved.
2. Family doctors in the area: they see most of the patients initially and will be a source of referrals.

3. Other practitioners: this will help you establish charges or fees for treatment. Undercutting is frowned upon and a greedy practitioner will soon gain an unenviable reputation.
4. The local branches of the major medical insurance companies: they will show you how the companies settle patients' accounts and the scale of fees they expect you to charge and for which they will pay.
5. If you have learned about a particular sport or dancing technique, then an approach to a local team or dance company may prove a source of interesting and rewarding work.

If you are unfamiliar with the area of the proposed practice, it is well worthwhile spending some time getting to know it and investigating opportunities for your practice. After all, when a move to a new part of the country is anticipated, enquiries are always made in respect of schools, shopping centres, leisure facilities, public transport and libraries. It is also helpful to have friends or relatives already established in the area, but failing any contacts, a personal approach and footwork is the only answer!

WHERE TO PRACTISE?

A practice in your home town

If you decide to practise in your home town, there is the satisfaction of contributing to the local community where you are known by friends and relatives; they may form the basis of instant referrals to the new practice, and the bank manager may be more ready to give you financial support.

There is, however, the old adage 'never mix business with pleasure', so the advantage of being well known and having friends in the locality may not benefit the practice as much as you think. Family and friends may be more critical than they would be of an unknown practitioner. On the other hand there may be a strong family tradition of medical practice in the area and this could be a great help in getting started.

Running a practice from home

This can be a very successful venture if the location, type of house and the profession you practise are all compatible.

It has many attractions. No time is spent travelling unless it is for domiciliary or hospital visits. If you practise from home it may be possible to allow a portion of the running costs of the house to be considered a tax deductable business expense, so you must consult your accountant for these financial implications.

However, it is not always possible to achieve an entirely professional atmosphere when working from home. It may be difficult to protect the patients from intrusions by the family or domestic matters; it may also be difficult to keep the family free from the inevitable changes the practice will bring into domestic routine. Space required by the practice will reduce the room available for private life. The undoubted advantages of practising from home need to be balanced against the wish to keep home quite separate from professional activities and have a retreat in which to relax.

Practising in premises

Premises may be bought, leased or rented and these alternatives are more fully discussed in Chapter 2.

1. *Purchased premises*

It can be argued that buying your own property is a wise financial move. There seems to be no end to the upward spiral of property values, and in your own premises you have the advantage of a steadily increasing asset. However, it may not always be possible to buy, either because the financial commitment is too great or the premises in which you want to practise are simply not for sale.

2. *Leasing*

This is probably the most popular method of acquiring premises and a good lease with well distanced rent review dates gives security without heavy capital commitment.

3. *Renting*

This is an option and it may be one which suits you. It does have certain disadvantages and, in general, it is probably safer to take a lease on premises than merely rent, as you will see in Chapter 2 where these alternatives are fully discussed.

In choosing the location for your practice, consider how far you need to travel. Travelling takes time, costs money and is very tiring.

It is not always the distance from home which may make premises undesirable, but the type of journey you will have to make. Driving 10 miles across central London in heavily congested traffic can take the best part of a frustrating hour or more, whereas 20 miles along a good motorway may be perfectly acceptable. One of the advantages of practising away from home is that professional and private life can be quite separate.

Domiciliary practice

It is necessary to treat and visit certain patients in their own homes. Team work between health professionals in a community is essential, and with the help of the patient's family and friends, domiciliary treatment can restore a patient to full health and independence.

Some practitioners, especially in remote rural areas or in a predominantly geriatric community, may find that a large part of their work is domiciliary. Patients are usually more seriously ill than those who can travel to the surgery or practice. Many have just been discharged from hospital and it is necessary for them to stay in their own homes.

Patients' homes vary as much as their conditions and they may not be as functional as your practice, so you will have to be adaptable. The following points may help:

1. Try not to travel great distances as it is expensive, time consuming and tiring.
2. Is your car suitable? How much petrol does it use per mile? How much does it cost to have it serviced? Are you using the family car? Is the car insured for business use? Do you have to carry expensive equipment or drugs in the car? Is equipment insured against wear and tear, vibration and theft? Are your drugs locked up and secure?
3. Can you detach yourself from the social implications of domiciliary work and preserve professional standards?
4. Can you cope with heavy patients, low beds, and the family behaviour in the home?
5. If you use electrical equipment, take extension cables and adaptors with you as power points are not universal.

Plan the route carefully with the aid of a reliable map. Treatment must be cost effective as time spent travelling to and from a practice costs money.

Domiciliary practice is a rewarding area of work and must be undertaken, not only on ethical and clinical grounds, but also in terms of practicality.

THE WAYS TO PRACTISE

When you commence private work you will need to decide which forms your practice will take. There are four main options:
1. Single-handed practice.
2. A partnership.
3. An association or group practice.
4. A limited company.

The freedom to choose may be restricted by legislation or the rules of your professional organisation. One of the characteristics of the human race is to organise into groups, and it is true that two heads can be better than one. But, whichever method is finally chosen will depend on your own physical and mental abilities, financial circumstances and personal aspirations. It need not be an irrevocable decision: you may decide to start working single-handed, and then meet a colleague with whom you feel you could work and form a partnership. All four methods have their advocates: it is up to you to determine and define your aims in order to find out what you really want.

Single-handed practice

The solo practitioner must be very independent, dedicated and confident. You are responsible for everything connected with the practice, including obtaining premises, fixtures and fittings, decoration, practice organisation, financial planning and management; and you will have to make all the decisions. Isolation can prove a little daunting, particularly if you have been working in a hospital where much of the support structure is provided and the responsibility is mainly clinical. However, you do have the satisfaction of knowing that the success of the practice is all your own work and, of course, the profits are entirely yours; but in the eyes of the law, a sole practitioner and the business are regarded as one, and it is not possible to claim that certain personal assets are distinguishable from any owned by the practice. This type of practice is very flexible: it can be set up without legal formality and the book-keeping requirements are fairly straightforward and simple. It gives great freedom, but it brings responsibility. Many practitioners enjoy working on their own and have highly successful and profitable practices.

The disadvantages occur when you are ill or you wish to take a holiday, for unless you close the practice or find a suitable locum, holidays become non-existent. If you are ill and cannot practise, there is no income.

Partnership

If you want shared responsibility, a partnership with one or more colleagues may be the answer. A partnership is preferably a formal legal relationship rather than an informal agreement with no legal authority.

A partnership consists of two or more people, who join together with a view to making a profit. The partnership is subject to certain legal formalities such as the sharing of profits. Each partner is personally liable for the debts of the partnership or of the individual partners if they are unable to meet their own debts. Therefore, there must be complete confidence and trust.

Partnerships have many advantages. Each partner may contribute capital and will devote time and energy to the success of the practice. Special skills and expertise may be complementary, thereby expanding the range of patients the practice can accept. Decisions, responsibilities and management of the practice will be shared. A partner may well bring in valuable referrals and contacts. In addition, an older and more experienced practitioner can be of considerable benefit to the practice.

A partner is invaluable if you are ill, have an accident or if you have to give time to a family crisis. Whether you personally are at work or not, the practice will continue, the patients will be seen and you are relieved of the worry of finding a colleague to cover for you while you are absent. Partners should not only be regarded as useful for the difficult times—it is also very pleasant to share success with somebody else and to plan for the future.

A partnership is, however, a close relationship and entails a great deal of tolerance and understanding if it is to be successful. A shared decision can mean one which is reached only through compromise and possibly argument. Disagreements are rarely over patients, but usually centre on management or financial matters. Patients identify with a particular partner and there is occasionally a cross-over during holidays, professional courses or sickness, so the attitudes and behaviour of the partners should convey an atmosphere of stability. Take your time over entering into a partnership. It may be a good idea to work together informally for a while to see how compatible you are before signing any agreements.

A partnership, whether informal or formal, is a social contract, and as in marriage, divorce can be expensive and upsetting. Partnership agreements are described in more detail in Chapter 4.

Association or group practice

An association is not ownership. Two or more practitioners join together to share expenses such as rent, rates, electricity and water charges. In this type of practice, therefore, you would have access to all the facilities, such as a receptionist, but remain independent, responsible for your patients and with complete control of your own finances. This option has many attractions, particularly the shared responsibility for the premises and facilities and the contact and friendship of fellow practitioners in your own and other professions. This can be very useful for referrals, on call duties and holiday arrangements.

Limited company

This is more complicated as it has an existence in law distinct from that of its owners. Shares will be issued and the business will have limited liability. The company will be responsible for all debtors, leases and other obligations that it takes upon itself. Unlike a partnership, it is possible to separate the assets and liabilities of the business so they are distinguishable from those of the owner or owners. The formation of a limited company is a complex matter and requires financial and legal advice. In some countries, there are restrictions imposed by the professional organisation on practitioners running a limited company, since it may contravene the rules of conduct. It is strongly suggested that advice is sought from the appropriate organisation if this step is contemplated (see the Appendix).

Entering private practice on a part-time basis

If ever an idea was open to individual interpretation, this is it. The concept of part-time may vary from seeing one or two patients a week outside a full-time National Health Service job to working almost full-time. The work may remain part-time or it can develop into a full-time commitment. One of the biggest headaches for the practitioner who has one or two private patients plus a permanent post, is what to do when the private practice side increases and the time to cope with it is just not available. When this happens, the decision as to whether or not to abandon the security of regular employment and take the step into full-time private practice work will have to be faced. It is true that the combination of job security and the pleasure of your own small private practice is irresistible: unfortunately, it is a difficult combination to maintain. Nevertheless, it is a very good way to 'see how the private work goes' and keep a steady income from permanent employment to pay for the essentials of life. There will, however, be certain tax implications which must be looked at thoroughly with an accountant when you are practising as an employee and have part-time self-employment. Some professional organisations do not approve of practitioners who are dividing their time and expertise. It is acceptable but is it possible to maintain the same quality of service when the two roles are combined?

As an assistant or locum

Working as an assistant in an already established practice can provide an ideal introduction to the clinical and managerial skills required for eventual ownership. Working in a well-organised and busy practice would help you build up your confidence and increase your skills. In time a partnership may be offered.

THE ADVANTAGES OF PRIVATE PRACTICE

Each individual will see the advantages differently, placing greater emphasis on one rather than the other. In general, the greatest advantage is considered to be the independence you will gain. Clearly nobody can live or work totally in isolation, but independence is a valuable asset. There is also the professional satisfaction of work well done, of being able to give sufficient time and attention to the patient, and the flexibility of the arrangements of the practice, such as hours of work.

Personal satisfaction will come from the self-discipline and effort needed to start and run a practice: the sense of achievement felt when, despite all the initial problems, you open your doors and begin a new and different phase of your life, will make it all seem worth it.

Hard work, enthusiasm and good professional patient care will bring a sense of pride and achievement which will more than justify the decision you make to start in private practice. Finally, it is you who will know why you wish to enter private practice, but test the market and have a keen awareness of costs before proceeding.

PRACTITIONER CHECK LIST

1. Do I know what private practice is?
2. Do I know how to approach the private practice sector?
3. Do I know who to approach?
4. Will I need to consult anyone else before entering private practice?
5. Am I in good health?
6. Have I discussed private practice with my family?
7. Do I want to leave my present employment?
8. Which form of practice should I consider?
9. Can I see all types of patients?
10. Do I need to specialise?
11. Have I considered all the ways of entering private practice?
12. Shall I proceed?

2

Starting in private practice

And gives to airy nothing
A local habitation and a name.
William Shakespeare 1564–1616

CHOOSING WHERE

It may take months of research and effort before the practitioner finds a location which is suitable for the practice. It will depend not only on finding acceptable premises or an existing practice, but also on finding an environment in which to enjoy a happy personal life and perhaps bring up a family.

Your first considerations in choosing where to practise must be geographical location and accessibility. It is also very important that the needs of the community and the practice opportunities match your personal, professional and financial requirements. The individual choice between a large city, a seaside town, the suburbs or a rural area will be influenced by these factors; and the place where you eventually practise will, to a certain extent, determine the pattern of the practice.

When you are deciding where to locate the practice, you might consider the following points:

The community's need for a practitioner

1. The number of other practitioners in the area.
2. What are their specialities?
3. Will the area support another practitioner?
4. What is the density of the population?
5. Is there anticipated growth or decline in the population?
6. Are medical resources widely used in the community?
7. Is it a city, a highly residential suburb, the country or primarily a commuter area?
8. What is the age group?
9. Are most people single, young married or elderly?
10. Is it a retirement area?

Personal needs and those of your family

1. Might the available property serve as a home and a practice (Fig. 2.1)?
2. What is the appearance of the property (Fig. 2.2)?
3. Are buildings or office premises available for purchase?
4. Will you lease or rent?

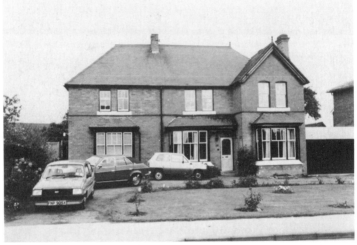

Fig. 2.1 A practice and a home (reproduced by kind permission of Mrs M. John MCSP).

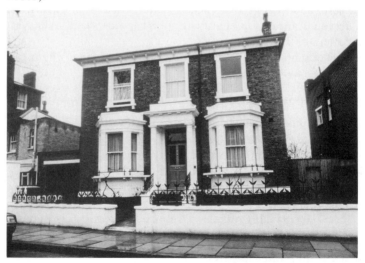

Fig. 2.2 A town practice (reproduced by kind permission of Mrs A. McLaughlin MCSP).

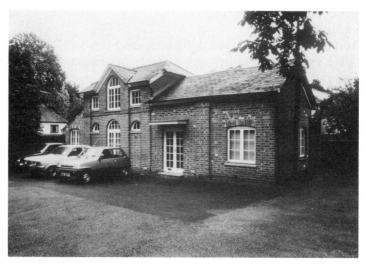

Fig. 2.3 A rural practice (reproduced by kind permission of Henley Physiotherapy Services).

5. Has the property plenty of car parking space (Fig. 2.3)?
6. Is there good access to public transport?
7. What are the recreational facilities and social opportunities?
8. Is there a good shopping centre?
9. Do you wish to practise in a busy high street or a remote rural area?
10. Is there a good garage in the vicinity? Car servicing and repairs are particularly important for domiciliary practice.
11. Are there good schools nearby? Will they suit the ages of your children?
12. How high are the local rates?
13. Is there more than one bank, a building society and a post office nearby?
14. Will the rest of the family be able to find work?
15. Will planning permission be necessary to convert the property for medical use?
16. Is there any likelihood of redevelopment in the area?
17. Are there any local licencing regulations relating to medical practice premises?

These last two points are discussed more fully later in this chapter.

The local medical facilities

Finally, the local medical community and any other services which may be needed for consultation and referral will have to be considered.

1. Is there a good local hospital or health centre?
2. What other practitioners are available for consultations and referral? Are they likely to be co-operative?
3. Does the professional organisation to which you belong have a local representative?
4. Are there opportunities for continuing post-registration education?
5. Is other clinical work available, for example, in sports centres, nursing homes and private clinics?
6. Is there a dispensing chemist in the area?
7. What fees are charged by other practitioners?
8. Are there any medical insurance company representatives in the region?

ACQUIRING PREMISES

There are various sources available to help you select suitable premises. You can advertise your requirements in the appropriate medical journals and periodicals, or in the local or national press. However, advertising can be expensive, and often just spreading the word that you are seeking some premises will produce results. Casual inquiries can seem vague, so be definite about your requirements and you will not miss an opportunity should it arise.

The estate agent

One of the most reliable ways of finding premises is to register with a reputable local estate agent. Tell him what you are looking for and the approximate location, and give him some idea of the price you can afford. He will give you invaluable help in identifying current local prices, rate levels and any local authority restrictions applying to a particular property. Try and be specific about your requirements, or you will find yourself deluged with information about every type of property, most of which will be totally unsuitable. This will waste a great deal of time. It is advisable to register with two or three agents so that you obtain as much information as possible, and therefore have a wider choice of available property.

If you are buying an existing practice or becoming a partner, an estate agent will probably help you in evaluating the property involved by giving some indication of the price you will have to pay.

The size and layout of the practice

It is vital to have a plan of how much space you require, and how the practice will be arranged. Try and work it out in terms of feet or metres as the property details from the estate agents will be set out in these terms.

A careful choice of space-saving equipment will make the most of small premises in an expensive location. You may have to compromise, but be careful. It is undesirable, for example, to have such a small reception area that patients are sitting on each other's knees! Modern buildings are often easier to convert and utilise than older ones, but with careful planning and sketches, maximum advantage can be gained from the available floor space (see Fig. 2.4).

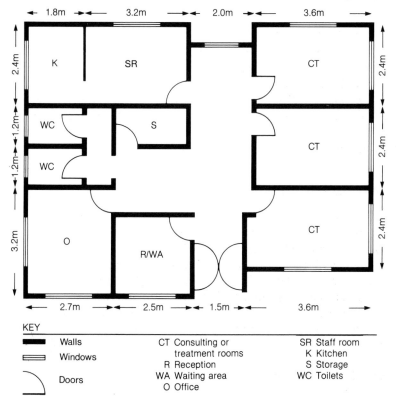

KEY

▬	Walls	CT	Consulting or treatment rooms	SR	Staff room
▭	Windows			K	Kitchen
		R	Reception	S	Storage
⌐	Doors	WA	Waiting area	WC	Toilets
		O	Office		

Fig. 2.4 Design layout to show proposed floor plan of a practice.

Moving is expensive and disruptive, so premises with sufficient space for expansion over the next few years are desirable. Larger premises can be a better long-term investment, as surplus accommodation can usually be sub-let until it is needed.

The architect

Anyone considering building a practice or extending existing premises, must seek help from an architect. It is wise to see as many designs as possible in operation, as this is the only way to check whether the architectural plans work in practice.

Estimates and quotations

It is advisable to have written estimates as a result of quotations from the builder, the decorator and any other service or company which may be required in setting up and equipping the practice. It gives you time to look at the costs and select the services you can afford before making any commitments.

Most companies will expect to be paid without delay, and will sometimes ask for a deposit or payment prior to delivery. This is inevitable if you are a new customer and have not yet established that you are worthy of credit.

Keep all the bills as they will provide a useful record for the future. Record the names of the people who have given a good service. It is easy to forget who did what and you may wish to use them again.

Time scale/factor

The first thing to bear in mind from the beginning is that everything, without exception, takes longer than you think.

Applications to local authorities can be very slow as the committees are very busy. They only meet on a regular basis, so if you miss one meeting, you may have to wait some time before the next one.

Any legal work tends to take a long time, particularly if there are more than two parties involved in the negotiations. This may be frustrating, but the solicitor is acting for you and will not wish to be hurried into making a mistake.

You can speed things up by always replying promptly to correspondence and by using the telephone if a letter is not essential.

The times listed in Figure 2.5 give you an idea of how long to wait for work to be done. The delays can be extremely annoying, as an empty property costs money. Commission all the work to go ahead promptly, so you are ready to see patients as soon as possible.

Fig. 2.5 A list of the approximate times that it may be necessary to allow before you start in private practice.

Time allowance	Item
1–2 weeks	Written estimates
6–8 weeks	Legal work
2–6 weeks	Telephone installation
6–12 weeks	Directory insertion
8–12 weeks	Planning permission
2–4 weeks	Printing requirements
2–6 weeks	Rewiring and decoration
1–4 weeks	Bank loan arrangements
2–4 weeks	Contacts with other practitioners and local hospitals
1–3 weeks	Accounting systems
3–6 months	The practice can start

PLANNING PERMISSION AND LOCAL AUTHORITIES

Before proceeding with the purchase of a freehold property or taking a lease, make sure that you are allowed to use it for medical practice. Many premises are designated for a particular use, such as for office or residential use only, and formal permission must be obtained for a change of use from the local authority. It may take from eight to twelve weeks for your application to come before the appropriate committee for consideration, and it may be turned down for any number of reasons such as: inadequate parking facilities, the building may have a conservation order on it, or it may be that the committee feel a medical practice in that particular location does not fit in with their planning or it does not comply with the Town and Country Planning Act 1976.

If permission is refused, it may be worth appealing against the decision in order to avoid losing suitable premises.

Permission may also have to be granted for professional nameplates to be displayed. If you alter the structure of the building substantially, the authority may want to view the plans and alterations to make sure that they are in accordance with local regulations.

Licences

In some countries it will be necessary to license the practice, but this varies according to the area, county or state in which you practise. Always check with the local authority and a solicitor to make sure that you are acting correctly. Legislation changes frequently, so it is wise to establish if anything new is relevant. The local authorities are often very helpful and may give a lot of useful advice.

Fire precautions

The local authorities will suggest that you contact the fire officer before you finally purchase a property. This is extremely wise for insurance purposes, as adequate fire precautions will not only protect your interests and property, but it is necessary to comply with certain regulations contained in the Health and Safety at Work Act 1974 and The Fire Precautions Act 1971. The fire officer will give advice on the provision of fire doors, the access to them, fire escapes and exits and the appropriate fire extinguishers which are described in Chapter 5.

THE PROPERTY

There are several points to consider when viewing a property and choosing premises, whether freehold or leasehold:
1. The structure, reputation and history of the building must enhance the professional image. A well-known address is worth a considerable amount.
2. What is the state of the decoration? Will painting be necessary?
3. Are the major services adequate and are they in good working order, for instance, safe electrical wiring, reliable plumbing with plenty of hot water? Replacing or repairing these items can be very expensive.
4. Is the property the right size and is it suitable for expansion?
5. Will planning permission be needed for structural alterations, such as an extension, or for change of use to medical premises?
6. Is it located in the right place for good access to public transport and are there car parking facilities to avoid congestion and annoyance to neighbours?

7. Is there a lift? This is important if the practice is not on the ground floor.
8. Is a ramp installation required?
9. Are there any long-term plans for the area, such as a by-pass, a block of flats or a new hospital?
10. Are there any restrictive covenants in the deeds?
11. If it is a leasehold property, what are the liabilities?
12. If it is a leasehold property, who is responsible for the external repairs?
13. Is there plenty of natural daylight?
14. Are the fire escapes and fire precautions up to the standard required and do they comply with the guidelines in the Health and Safety at Work Act 1974. (See Bibliography, The Law on Health and Safety at Work, p. 153.)
15. Is there plenty of storage space? You always need more than you think.
16. Is the property divided by partitions or has it solid walls?
17. Is it reasonably quiet?
18. Are the neighbours or other users of the building quiet and tidy?

Most of these points can easily be ascertained by the estate agent: it will save a lot of time to have all the queries to hand, so you can get them answered before proceeding.

Any questions the estate agent cannot answer will be clarified by a solicitor, who will carry out searches on the property and the surrounding area before you sign any contract.

Freehold property

It is not easy to estimate the current market value of freehold property, especially if you are a stranger to the area. So do take the advice of a reliable estate agent and a surveyor: their skill and judgement will be invaluable.

The final purchase must be suitable for your professional and personal requirements, the price must be right and, ideally, the property will be free from any restrictions in respect of alteration or use. The purchase of a freehold property will also represent an increasingly valuable asset. This is important as one day you may wish to move and sell it. There are certain tax implications if you purchase a property as a home and intend to use part of it as a practice, and these are described in Chapter 3.

If your home is also a practice or surgery, check that the

neighbours will not object to the subsequent increase in traffic or the medical practice itself.

The purchase of a freehold property, therefore, represents a major financial commitment, and personal circumstances will determine whether it is a step to be taken.

Leasehold property

By taking a lease on a property, you will save on an initial capital outlay, although you will have to pay a premium for the lease. Rent is payable at quarterly intervals in advance and is reviewed periodically, every three or five years, the rent remaining the same between reviews.

At the end of the lease, which is normally ten to fifteen years, the tenant is protected by certain provisions in the Landlord and Tenant Act 1954 Part II which governs business tenancies. For example, the tenant has a right to extend the lease if he wishes on the same terms as the old lease, except in certain circumstances in Section 24 of the Act, for example if the landlord wishes to occupy the premises himself. Reading and understanding a lease is not easy and it is essential a solicitor goes through it with you, so that you know what you are entitled to under its terms and what your responsibilities and obligations are.

You must try and establish an amicable relationship with the landlord as there may be terms in the lease which you may wish to change and for which you need his agreement. All landlords want a satisfied tenant. If you are helpful to him, he will co-operate with you. It may well be that the building is owned by a large company who have appointed a firm of managing agents to look after their interests. Generally, these firms are very helpful in meeting reasonable requirements and requests. It is worth getting to know the agent responsible for your building as it makes it easier to ask for what you want.

You must also establish with the landlord or managing agents that you can put a professional nameplate on the exterior of the building.

Renting a property

When you rent premises, there is generally no written agreement between tenant and landlord. There is no protection of tenure and no way of compelling the landlord to carry out any of his obligations. It can be considered an insecure way to practise. However, it is possible to rent space from another practitioner and this informal arrangement may well be satisfactory for a short time.

PURCHASING AN EXISTING PRACTICE

Buying property which is already an existing practice is not as elementary as it may seem from the 'For Sale' notices appearing in the professional journals or periodicals. The practice may be in a freehold, leased or rented property, and there are certain very important questions that must be asked, as buying will involve a considerable capital outlay.

Why is the practice for sale?

This is the first question you must ask. There will probably be perfectly legitimate reasons and possibly more doubtful ones:
1. Ill health or retirement of the practitioner.
2. Death of the previous practitioner.
3. The vendor is moving elsewhere.
4. Family commitments.
5. The premises may be poorly located with consequent low patient attendance.
6. The expiration of the lease has occurred. It may be renewable but only at an unacceptable and uneconomic rent.
7. There are proposals to alter the area around the practice (for example, with a one-way system which will prevent easy access by car, a motorway or the construction of an undesirable institution).

These last three points must make you extremely cautious over any decision to purchase. On the other hand, plans for a new housing development, a sports club, or a new school, will obviously be advantageous.

Unless the reason is obvious, such as ill health or retirement, the vendor does not have to say why the practice is for sale. It is up to you to find out. Do not forget: the vendor knows a great deal more about the practice than you do, and he may try to conceal facts which could deter a prospective purchaser. It takes a very discerning eye to see a shaky structure behind an impressive facade. However, most practices are sold for quite genuine reasons with the vendor only too willing to co-operate in every way in order to complete a successful and quick sale.

What is for sale?

The initial advertisement will indicate whether the practice is a single-handed one or a partnership, or whether an associate is required to join a group practice.

The type of property, i.e. whether it is freehold, leasehold or rented, and the amount of space and facilities, will be specified in the advertisement. Details of fixtures and fittings and any equipment to be sold will also be included. The asking price will sometimes be given, but this may well be open to negotiation according to the assets and the condition of the practice.

A great deal of time can be wasted in going to see practices which fail to live up to expectations, so try and find out as many details as possible before you take the time and the trouble to make a visit.

Scrutinising the practice finances

Accounts must be available for all the years the practice has been in operation. These will show the financial state of the practice. The accounts will exhibit how much income has been generated, what the expenses and overheads are, and what the profit was. They will show whether the practice is expanding or whether it has reached a certain point and levelled off.

It is an obvious danger sign if the vendor cannot produce any accounts for a period ending in the last eighteen months. One year's accounts are not sufficient to show the true financial position, so be careful. It may be difficult to understand the figures and terms used by accountants, so have them explained to you.

The accounts may, for example, conceal opportunities such as an undervalued property or under-estimated values for fixtures and fittings.

Evaluating the assets

The assets are tangible commodities gained in exchange for the purchase price.

1. *The property*

The property itself is an investment. If you are buying a freehold property, then this will be an increasingly attractive and valuable asset. It is also one which is most readily saleable or which can be used as security if you need to borrow money.

If you are purchasing a lease or a leasehold property, then this too will represent an asset if you wish to move during the term of the lease and sell it to another practitioner.

The condition, location and general appearance of the property must be assessed and valued by a reputable surveyor. The cost of essential alterations, repairs or decorations will, therefore, add to the eventual purchase price.

2. The equipment

This must be correctly valued. It may be in need of repair, old or obsolete. It could, however, be brand new, modern and just what you want. The value of equipment may be perceived very differently by the parties involved. The vendor may see it as perfectly workable, well loved and totally adequate. The purchaser, however, may not be able to imagine ever using any of it! A compromise on its value will be inevitable. Depreciation in the value of the equipment will show in the accounts as can be seen in Chapter 3.

The current price of the equipment can be assessed by an engineer or a representative of the manufacturing company who supplied it.

3. The stock

This is medical supplies and office stationery. The stock will be easy to value as current prices will be readily available, and an itemised stock list, together with a realistic assessment of its value, is essential, in case it is outdated and needs replacing.

4. Debtors

The question whether patients who have outstanding bills at the time of the sale of the practice are going to pay, and if so, when, has to be asked of the vendor. This may well be an asset which you can do without. It is necessary to obtain a warranty from the vendor, or to discount the debtors from the eventual purchase price of the practice.

5. Fixtures and fittings

A word of warning about the fixtures and fittings: whatever you may feel about them, try not to be condemnatory. These items have been part of the vendor's professional life, probably for some years. A few badly chosen remarks at any stage could jeopardise the sale. The vendor may wish to argue over details, but do not revise any firm conclusions you may have about them. Patience and tact will help you reach a satisfactory compromise.

6. *Records*

Patients' notes have to be meticulously kept, maintained and stored safely for some years. These are essential for reference in the future and will show the number of treatments or consultations, and the subsequent cash flow. The number of domiciliary patients must be noted since they represent the time spent away from the practice which is expensive, and therefore not always an asset.

7. *Goodwill*

What is goodwill? It is notoriously hard to identify but is an asset of the practice, albeit an intangible one, for which you will have to pay. Accountants use the term quite specifically to cover an array of items which cannot be put under any other heading when it comes to preparing the accounts, and may not put a figure on it.

The vendor uses the term rather more specifically to cover:

a. The medical contacts and referral system with other practitioners. These will have been established over many years and will be passed on to you.
b. The reputation and success of the practice.
c. The loyalty of the patients.
d. The fact that patients and practitioners know the practice telephone number.
e. Good relationships with trades people and medical suppliers.

It cannot be assumed, however, that the vendor's goodwill will stay with the purchasing practitioner. Will the patients or professional colleagues continue to trust the practice and use your services or will they go elsewhere? Will the contract the vendor has with the local nursing home remain with the practice or will it be passed on to somebody else?

The balance that is finally struck between the figure for which the vendor is prepared to sell and that which the purchaser is prepared to pay over and above the value of the other assets, is goodwill. The amount you pay will be eventually reconciled as a matter of agreement and negotiation between both parties with the advice of an accountant.

Goodwill cannot qualify for tax deduction for either the vendor who is selling an existing practice or the purchaser. It is considered as a capital item and is not included in the taxable income.

It will benefit the vendor to have the price of the goodwill as high as possible to reduce the possibility of incurring tax on the profit of the sale of the assets of the practice. The purchaser will want the price of the assets to be high, as it will constitute the cost price for depreciation purposes.

There are various formulae for calculating the amount of goodwill, such as a percentage of the average gross income over the previous three years, or the number of patients per year multiplied by the current fee that the practice is charging and the number of domiciliary visits. It is a matter of individual choice and negotiation between the vendor and the purchaser who have to reach a compromise with the help of their accountants.

8. *Staff*

An efficient, happy staff is one of the most important assets of an established practice. It is essential to minimise any uncertainty or rumour arising from the practice changing hands in order to avoid loss of key staff whom you may be very anxious to retain. Do not, however, make any commitments which cannot be kept if the staff should subsequently prove unsuitable.

Negotiating the price

Having studied the accounts, evaluated the assets and taken the advice of an accountant and a solicitor, you can make an offer to buy the practice in the region of the asking price. The vendor may have a firm price in mind. It will probably be higher than that which you are prepared to pay. Negotiations over the price will continue until an agreeable amount is reached. Do not forget that the vendor is selling what may be a lifetime's work and interest. It will be a difficult time for him, so have patience.

Any negotiation has a natural time span and it is an instinctive skill to determine that time and then reach a firm conclusion on the price.

Paying for the practice

This is described in Chapter 3. A good forecast of the practice potential will be available and if you are not in the happy position of having the cash to pay for the practice outright, which is extremely rare, then you will have to seek a source of finance.

The advantages of buying

These can be numerous, even though you have to make changes which can be time consuming and frustrating.

The advantages are:

1. You are buying an existing practice and hopefully a thriving business or at least one with potential. In effect, you are taking over a number of patients and the assets immediately, which will help establish the practice financially.
2. The practice will already have a telephone, which will save having to organise a new installation, and the number will be familiar to patients and practitioners alike.
3. Fixtures and fittings are *in situ*. They may not be entirely to your own taste, but you can change them gradually.
4. The equipment may be perfectly adequate for your use, and as it becomes obsolete, you can change it.
5. The practice will be established and known. This will be a great advantage, especially in the early days when you are getting started.

A note of caution

The premises you choose for the practice is an individual decision. You will have to sign some form of agreement or contract. Do take advice before you sign. Mistakes can be expensive so make sure you are getting what you want. Hasten slowly. Recognise the problems and use the help and information of the professional advisers, and the vendor, to allow negotiations to proceed smoothly. However, an ancient note of warning: *Caveat emptor* (Let the buyer beware).

PROFESSIONAL ADVISERS

The importance of the roles played by an accountant and a solicitor cannot be over-emphasised. You are going to use their advice and help quite frequently, so it is important they are chosen carefully.

Do not necessarily select the one nearest to the practice, and it is unwise to go to someone you know only in a social capacity since he is going to know all your details and problems.

When to look for an accountant

Do not delay in seeking an accountant; it is the first and most important step. He is not a luxury. He is essential if you are going to avoid a great deal of paperwork. His expertise in managing various forms and documents related to tax matters will be invaluable. You do not have the necessary skill and knowledge to cope with this on your own. Tax concessions may be lost without proper advice, and once information has been given to the tax authorities, it is often not possible to alter the information at a later stage, even if this results in an unfavourable tax situation at a later date. Proposed trading figures, overheads and cash flow for the first year can roughly be estimated with the accountant's help once all the figures and written estimates have been established. This will assist you when you first visit the bank manager.

If, due to financial pressure, a part-time National Health appointment is retained until the new practice is self-supporting, then the tax situation will be more complex, as is described in Chapter 3.

The accountant

The accountant will be responsible for the following:
1. Setting up and monitoring the financial record keeping.
2. Establishing sound financial guidelines on expenditure, salaries and pensions.
3. Advising on, analysing and projecting the growth and development of the practice.
4. Preparing the annual balance sheet and income statement.
5. Dealing with all tax matters.

The solicitor

A solicitor is another necessary adviser. You must ask his advice in connection with all legal matters. Lease agreements, conveyance documents, partnership, limited company and insurance agreements must all be seen by him. Make sure he has a good reputation and if you do not have a family solicitor, take the steps that are suggested below.

Where to look for an accountant and solicitor

If you do not already have an accountant or family solicitor, the recommendation of a friend or another practitioner may help you find them.

Other sources for help are:

1. The manager of the bank or finance company.
2. The professional organisation of whichever adviser you are seeking. The relevant addresses are listed in the Appendix.
3. The Yellow Pages of the local telephone directory.
4. The Citizen's Advice Bureau.
5. The public library.

You may find an adviser who is working at home and will offer his services to help you start. Alternatively, it is wise to choose someone who has the specialised knowledge of the self-employed practitioner, plus the ability and competence to apply it effectively.

A small practice with two or three partners may be the most suitable. It will be easier to establish rapport and trust with your adviser and, most important, if he is away or ill, one of the other partners will be able to help you if there is an urgent query or emergency.

Large firms are best avoided. They will offer a range of highly specialised services which you probably do not need, and the cost of these services will be reflected in their charges to you.

Fees

Make sure you have the scale of fees of your advisers clarified before going ahead. They are often calculated on a 'time occupied basis', with the hourly rate varying for the level of expertise of the staff required to carry out the work related to your practice affairs.

The insurance broker

The insurance broker is another very important person, as you will need several different types of insurance in both your personal and professional life. Insurance is a minefield for the inexperienced. It is a highly complex, diverse, confusing and competitive market. The expertise of a reputable broker is vital as you cannot afford to be inadequately insured in private practice. Insurances are discussed more fully in Chapter 4, but a list of the types of insurance you will need is given here for guidance:

1. Professional liability insurance.
2. Employer's liability insurance.
3. Public liability insurance.
4. Insurance for the practice and its contents.
5. Consequential loss insurance.
6. Private health insurance.
7. Permanent health insurance.
8. Pension and retirement insurance.
9. Car insurance for both personal and business use.
10. Insurance to cover mortgage payments.
11. Household insurance, that is, your house and its contents.
12. Computer insurance.

There are a vast number of policies on the market, each apparently offering slightly different cover. Do not take a policy and hope it will be suitable. Make sure it is what you want and give the broker all the material facts.

The bank manager

A sympathetic and helpful bank manager is essential in financing the initial capital expenditure and providing you with a reserve to pay continuing expenses until the practice begins to generate some income.

It is a good idea to have a talk with him before you begin looking for premises or take the first steps towards starting a private practice. He then knows what you have in mind and can advise you on a number of matters. He may even put you in touch with the other professional people who may be of help to you.

The bank manager will tell you the best method of obtaining credit. It may be a loan or overdraft facilities, or it may be a business loan with a pre-determined pay back arrangement on a monthly basis. These methods are all described in the next chapter in much greater detail, as are other sources from which you may wish to obtain the initial capital.

Banks, on the whole, are kindly disposed towards applications for professional practice facilities. Small branches of the major high street clearing banks do have limited overdraft and loan facilities, and may have to refer requests for large amounts of money to the head office. Therefore, it is wise to choose a bank and a manager who can finance both your anticipated and unforeseen expenditures. Unless there is a serious problem, you will have no difficulty in obtaining the money you need for the practice.

PRACTITIONER CHECK LIST

1. Where will I practice:
   in the town?
   in the country?
2. Do I want to live on the practice premises?
3. Have I planned how much space I will need?
4. Do I need planning permission?
5. Do I need a licence to practise?
6. Have I seen the fire officer to discuss precautions?
7. Have I arranged for the services of an accountant, a solicitor, and a banker?
8. Have I checked the lease with a solicitor?
9. Do I know how much space will suffice for five years?
10. Will it be necessary to make alterations to the building?
11. Is there good access, light, drainage, parking facilities etc.?
12. Have I seen accounts for at least the last three years of the practice I am purchasing?
13. Have I had estimates for all the work to be done?
14. Have I really decided which type of property is the most suitable?
15. Do I understand the meaning of 'goodwill'?
16. Am I ready to start?

3

Financial planning and management

There are few ways in which a man can be more innocently employed than in getting money.
Samuel Johnson 1709–1784

RUNNING A BUSINESS

Private practice is a business and in order to survive, it is necessary to make a PROFIT.

This chapter is intended to help the practitioner understand the basics of financial planning and management. It describes some of the methods used in the United Kingdom, although many of the principles will be applicable wherever you practise. If you wish to be successful, it is advisable to become familiar with the terms used in book-keeping and to be able to read financial statements.

You cannot afford to be ignorant or careless with figures since you will have to evaluate the clinical work and relate it to the financial position of the practice.

Every practice will require an investment of capital and you must be convinced that the future benefit is worth the investment risk.

You cannot run a business without financial control and private practice is no different from any other business. You are going to have onerous responsibilities. Are you skilled enough to justify the time and money involved in private practice? In order to find out, you must plan.

PLANNING

Everyone has to make a plan or budget at some time in order to produce better results. A business plan will help you assess and define your objectives and will help you to reach your goals. You will have to examine what is happening in the medical service in your area of practice in order to see the market variations and to identify your opportunities for future expansion.

The short-term plan

You must assess how much finance you will need for the first year. The day-to-day running costs of the practice must be carefully thought out and written down. This cannot be done quickly. You will need to obtain full details and estimates from any outside advisers you are using and this takes time. You will need CAPITAL to finance the practice. There are two kinds of capital.

1. *Initial capital*

This is the money which will be used to set up the practice, and purchase the property, the fixtures and fittings and any new medical equipment or stocks. This capital outlay is for items which are known as fixed assets; it is also used for replacing outdated equipment or purchasing a car.

2. *Working capital*

This is the money needed to finance the running of the practice. It is for the day-to-day costs, such as salaries, rates, insurance, bank charges, laundry, heat, light and water. The money spent on these overheads comes from the fees paid to you by your patients. It is referred to as revenue expenditure. Surplus revenue which is not used to cover these costs will become the profit of the practice.

The long-term plan

Having achieved the first year in practice, a pattern of expenditure and income will emerge and the potential of the practice will become evident. Are you making a profit? Has the original short-term plan worked? Can future plans be improved to provide more accurate results? It may become clear that the work load is too heavy for you to carry out on your own, and you may wish to expand and develop.

You will then have to consider the following points:
1. Do I need to employ staff?
2. Shall I extend the premises to accommodate extra patients?
3. Is there a demand for some sort of specialisation which might, therefore, give a higher turnover of patients?
4. Will it be necessary to purchase more equipment?

You plan for results, and although there must be some degree of flexibility in the planning of the practice, it is important to try and stick to a reasonably well defined set of goals and to try and achieve them within the time you have allowed. Like many things in life, the plan does not always work out as hoped. It is sometimes difficult to estimate the costs for the first year. It is usual for a new business to incur expenses which have not been anticipated. As a general principle, you should always over-estimate your costs.

It is advisable to keep the plan simple in the first year: assess what you have, what you need to borrow and keep any purchases to a minimum, especially when buying stock.

Obviously there are risks along the way, but with care and cautious optimism, you will survive.

ESTABLISHING COSTS

At the beginning you will have to estimate the following costs. It pays to take time and trouble over this as the variations from your estimates will be vitally important in all future decisions:

Setting up costs

These costs can be substantial. Make sure your list is as comprehensive as possible because the information you provide will help the accountant prepare a cash flow statement. This is necessary when you make an approach to a bank manager, finance company or any other source, to borrow money.

The following points can be used as a check-list of the items to plan for and organise:

1. The cost of buying, leasing or renting the premises. The purchase of the practice will be the largest item and will vary according to the location, size and type of practice you have chosen.
2. The cost of any alterations, repairs to the plumbing or heating, electrical work and any decoration. Obtain several estimates from reputable firms. It is not always wise to choose the cheapest as the work and service may not be very good.
3. Any office furniture, medical equipment and supplies must be costed. Initially, these will only be essential items. It is not cost effective to have pieces of expensive equipment that are only used occasionally, gathering dust and using up floor space. Do research thoroughly to find out what items you need and the best available prices.

4. The printing and stationery costs, which will include the letterheads, a possible logo and the doorplate.
5. The cost of all the linen, pillows, blankets, towels and professional clothing.
6. Fire, safety and security precautions must be costed. Enlist the help of a fire appliances company and a good locksmith.
7. A car if you do not already own one.
8. Essential medical reference books and journals.

All these items of capital expenditure become the tangible assets of the practice.

Running costs

Once the setting up costs and initial capital expenditure have been determined, you must establish the day-to-day costs of running the practice. These costs will include the following:

1. The annual outgoings, such as rates on property, the services charges on the premises if leased, and electricity, water and gas.
2. Car repairs and servicing.
3. Postage and stationery.
4. Professional subscriptions, periodicals and medical journals.
5. Travelling expenses for the business.
6. Telephone charges.
7. If there are to be staff, the cost of their salaries, your share of their National Insurance contributions and any benefits. Some guidelines can be obtained from either other practitioners or the professional organisation.
8. Accountancy and legal charges.
9. Insurances premiums.
10. Cleaning and laundry.

Hidden costs

Hidden costs do not remain hidden once the bills start to arrive!

1. If you are moving house, allow for the cost of actually moving. It can be very expensive, so obtain some written estimates well ahead of time. It is unfortunately not a business allowable expense.
2. Although accountancy and legal charges have been mentioned, you may have interim bills for which you have not estimated. These will be for the preparatory advice and help which the accountant and solicitor have given you. It is, therefore, wise to

establish whether they are asking for a few hundred pounds or a few thousand.

3. You must also include any provision for loan or overdraft interest and repayment.
4. National Insurance contributions must be remembered.
5. Tax provision is often forgotten. You must put aside sufficient money each month to cover the projected tax bill. It can be put in an interest-bearing account, such as a deposit or building society account. When you have to pay tax, the money is already set aside and a payment of a lump sum from your current account will not be necessary; you also have the added advantage of gaining a little interest in the meantime.

Personal needs

It is important to make a list of your personal needs as they will determine the amount of money you will draw out of the practice. In the first instance, you cannot rely on this amount being as high as your previous earnings, so allow for this.

Some of the items you will need to cover in your personal day-to-day expenses are:

1. Food and related items.
2. Personal clothing.
3. The hairdresser.
4. School fees.
5. Entertainment and holidays.
6. Personal transport.
7. Personal insurance.
8. A mortgage.

You will have to be careful with such items as clothing as only a certain proportion will be regarded as a business expense.

Costing your fees

The fees for each patient cannot be analysed specifically as they will depend on the condition of the patient and how much time is going to be spent in assessing, examining, prescribing for and treating the patient. Surgery may be involved which will require specialised skills and more time.

Having worked out as far as possible what your expenditure is going to be in the first year and how much capital may be required, you will now have to establish how you are going to cover it by the fees received from the patients. On a simple basis, it is necessary to estimate how many patients you can see each day and ascertain the fees that are going to be charged.

The quality of the services you offer is an indication of your professional skills. The hours of work must be arranged at a price high enough to ensure the recovery of all the salaries, overheads and expenses and to allow an even cash flow and an acceptable profit. Setting fees is one of the areas of private practice which is always talked around but never talked about. You have to get the fees right and the following points may help you:

1. The complexity of the patient's problem.
2. The skill, work and specialised knowledge involved in caring for the patient.
3. The time spent with the patient.
4. The number of letters and medical reports which have to be prepared.
5. The number of telephone calls which have to be made.

In addition:

6. Other practitioners will give some indication of fees in the area.
7. The major medical insurance companies may be able to help also by indicating their scale of charges and what fees are usual in your region.
8. The professional organisation usually has guidelines about fees.

You cannot plan a budget and cash flow system until the fees are established. Do not undervalue your services. Being professional means putting the right price on your efforts and the hours you work.

It is essential to calculate the number of patients and treatments which will cover your costs. This will depend on the fee structure you choose and the ratio of domiciliary and practice appointments.

Example

Let us assume that your average weekly expenditure is £750.00. You will, therefore, have to see ten patients a day at the minimum fee of £15.00 per session to cover the costs. If a charge of £16.00 per session is made, you will make a small profit.

BUDGETING AND FORECASTING

Once the total running costs have been calculated and the estimated income from patients' fees has been established, it will be possible to draw up a projected income and expenditure statement. Figure 3.1 is a statement setting out the running costs against the cash

	£	£
Income		
Fees charged for treatment		48,000
Expenses		
Salaries	16,300	
Loan interest	1,000	
Rates and water	2,500	
Lighting and heating	300	
Telephone	500	
Laundry and cleaning	1,000	
Motor and travelling expenses	1,200	
Repairs and engineer services	150	
Insurance	200	
Accountancy and legal fees	800	
Postage and stationery	500	
Medical sundries	3,800	
Office sundries	650	
Subscriptions	100	
Depreciation	1,000	
		30,000
EXCESS OF INCOME OVER EXPENDITURE (i.e. Profit for the year)		£18,000

Fig. 3.1 Projected income and expenditure statement.

income; this statement will be extremely helpful when you visit the bank manager for the first time to borrow money.

A profit and loss account

This account sets out the fees earned and the expenditure of the practice, the difference being the profit of the practitioner or the partners.

Budgeting

Budgeting is the process of estimating your income as it is earned and the expenditure as it is incurred. It will be obvious that this is a timing system and different from cash flow.

Cash flow

The cash flow statement sets out what is happening in cash terms. It tabulates the money going out of the practice to pay for expenses, and the money coming in. The outgoing expenses sometimes have to be settled when there is no money coming in from fees. This is a cash flow problem. The great majority of patients do not settle their accounts immediately at the end of a period of treatment and many do not pay until a long time after. Therefore, although there may be potential cash in the bank, until it is actually in the account it cannot be part of the cash flow.

A word of warning here, at certain periods of the year there are going to be heavy expenses, and in the beginning these will be numerous. Some will not be continuous, such as decorating or carpeting the premises, but others, such as telephone charges and car expenses, will continue. On quarter days, when the electricity bill, the insurance premium and the telephone account can all arrive within a few days of each other, payment will seriously deplete the account. Try to allow for these periods by putting aside money to meet these expenses and pay bills on the day you are obliged to.

At certain times the practice will be quiet, and therefore the income from fees will be low. This is a time to work hard at strict credit control which is described in Chapter 6.

Every business experiences ups and downs in expenses and income, so careful forecasting is essential, and it is advisable to always allow a margin for inflation in the forthcoming year.

Figure 3.2 is a simplified cash flow statement.

	Jan.	Feb.	Mar.	Apr.	May	June	July	Aug.	Sept.	Oct.	Nov.	Dec.
Initial expenditure												
Furniture & fittings	1,500											
Motor car	3,600											
Equipment	2,600											
Stocks	350											
	8,050											
Drawings required	1,000	1,000	1,000	1,000	1,000	1,000	1,000	1,000	1,000	1,000	1,000	1,750
Business expenditure	1,850	2,000	2,000	2,500	2,500	2,500	2,500	2,500	2,500	2,500	2,500	2,500
TOTAL PAYMENTS	10,900	3,000	3,000	3,500	3,500	3,500	3,500	3,500	3,500	3,500	3,500	4,250
Receipts	—	1,000	2,000	3,500	5,000	5,000	5,000	5,000	5,000	5,000	5,000	5,000
Surplus/(deficit) for month	£(10,900)	(2,000)	(1,000)	—	1,500	1,500	1,500	1,500	1,500	1,500	1,500	750
Accumulative cash surplus/(deficit)	£(10,900)	(12,900)	(13,900)	(13,900)	(12,400)	(10,900)	(9,400)	(7,900)	(6,400)	(4,900)	(3,400)	(2,650)

Cash summary to year end

Bank overdraft per balance sheet	6,900
Deduct: Deposit account	6,250
Net cash deficit	650
Capital introduced	2,000
Net cash outgoings per cash flow	£2,650

Fig. 3.2 Simplified cash flow statement.

The balance sheet

The final accounting item with which you will have to become familiar for budgeting and forecasting, is the balance sheet (see Fig. 3.3). It shows what the practice is worth. It is usually set out at the end of the practice's financial year, showing what the practice owns and what it owes.

Learning to read a balance sheet is important, especially if you intend purchasing an existing practice when you will wish to look at the accounts for at least the previous three years.

1. *Fixed assets*

These are the items that are permanently necessary for the practice to function, such as medical equipment, a car, premises, fixtures and fittings.

2. *Current assets*

These are assets from which cash will be realised in the current course of business, usually considered to be one year. Debtors, the value of any stock and the cash you have in the bank are all current assets.

3. *Fixed or long-term liabilities*

These liabilities do not have to be repaid immediately, so they become 'fixed'. These are such items as a long-term loan.

Current liabilities

Interest on a loan which has to be paid promptly comes under the heading current liabilities. Any sums of money which you owe to suppliers are also current liabilities.

Forecasting

Forecasting will show how much income you must take to break even and then start to make a profit.

Problems will occur because:
1. You have not paid enough attention to future cash requirements.
2. You have not enough information about the cost of the service you are providing. Are your fees correct?

	£	£
FIXED ASSETS		
Fixtures and fittings	1,500	
Less: Depreciation	150	
	———	1,350
Motor car	3,600	
Less: Depreciation	600	
	———	3,000
Medical equipment	2,600	
Less: Depreciation	250	
	———	2,350
		———
		6,700
CURRENT ASSETS		
Stock	350	
Deposit account	6,250	
Debtors for fees	1,500	
	———	8,100
		———
		14,800
DEDUCT: CURRENT LIABILITIES		
Bank loan account	6,900	
Creditors	650	
	———	7,550
		———
Net worth		£7,250
REPRESENTED BY:		
Capital introduced		2,000
Profit for year	18,000	
Less: Drawings	12,750	
	———	5,250
		———
PROPRIETORS INVESTMENT		£7,250

Note: Taxation on profits is ignored for this exercise

Fig. 3.3 Balance sheet at year end.

3. Your credit control is not strict enough. Are debtors paying their accounts?
4. Your inventory control of medical supplies is not being monitored sufficiently?

It is necessary to employ some method of being accurate: this can be done in the following way:

a. Forecast the total fees and interest for the year, distinguishing between the different types of work.
b. Forecast the total expenditure for the year; divide it into monthly averages with specific headings.
c. Keep monthly records of both fees and expenses to see whether forecasts are being achieved.
d. Use a time costing system as a means of directly controlling results.

Break-even chart

When you have arrived at the costs which are relatively fixed, you can predict the effect of your decisions on profitability. A simple example of a break-even chart (see Fig. 3.4) will show you when you are starting to make a profit.

1. The fixed costs are those which have to be paid whether there are any patients or not.
2. The variable costs are the costs producing the service, which vary according to the fee income. In a stable private practice, these costs are small and can usually be ignored.
3. The direct costs are your work and any medical supplies or equipment which are used to treat the patient.

Number of treatments

Calculate the number of treatments or fees on a fee income report chart (see Fig. 3.5). This will demonstrate monthly fluctuations, which will depend on the fee structure and the ratio between practice, hospital and domiciliary visits.

If the chart is kept on a noticeboard in the office, it will provide encouragement for you and your staff, enabling you to see where alterations, holidays and problems are occurring in the practice.

Staff

If you are deciding whether to employ additional staff, such as a

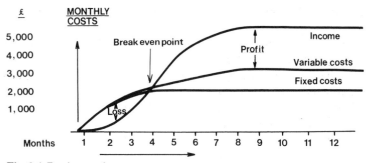

Fig. 3.4 Break even chart.

receptionist or an assistant, it will be necessary to forecast and determine the following points:
1. What effect will additional staff have on projected fees.
2. What effect will additional staff have on projected expenses.
3. In view of the present position of the practice, and its future, is it advisable to take on staff?

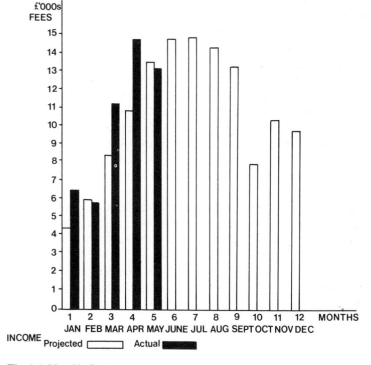

Fig. 3.5 Monthly fee income report.

It will become obvious that the profit and loss account, the balance sheet and forecasting and budgeting are extremely necessary as valuable indicators of the economic state of the practice. The information will be required by Her Majesty's Inspector of Taxes, and it will assist the bank manager and the manager of any other source of finance in advising you on your current and proposed financial requirements and in determining whether to lend you the money.

SOURCES OF FINANCE

Having planned and projected your cash flow and budget, there are plenty of sources with money available. It is waiting to be put to good use, providing you make the approach in the right way.

There are several methods of raising money which will depend on your personal circumstances. Some of these are direct forms of borrowing, such as an overdraft, or obtaining a longer-term loan.

Most self-employed people, small businesses and often limited companies, borrow from one of the major banks, but this is by no means the only source of finance.

Savings

You may have personal money which is in a building society, a deposit account, or invested in stocks and shares. The decision whether to use savings to obviate or at least reduce the amount of money you have borrowed is not an easy one to make.

Many people like to feel they have something in reserve for the proverbial rainy day, and therefore they keep their savings intact. If your money is wisely invested, it will be accumulating interest, so it is probably sensible to leave it where it is. However, most banks will require a contribution from personal savings, as they will be reluctant to finance the total requirements.

Approaching the bank

The manager in the local high street bank, which is probably a branch of one of the major clearing banks, is the most convenient and immediate person to approach for finance. He will try to help you, since lending money is an important part of his business. He will want to know what you are hoping to do and the opportunities which are going to make the practice a success. Go well prepared with the information he requires and anticipate a series of questions.

The main questions will be as follows:

1. Why do you want the money?
2. How much do you want?
3. How will the money be repaid?
4. What securities are being offered against any loan or overdraft?
5. What are the risks?

The bank manager needs to know that he can safeguard the money he may advance and that you will use it well. This also applies if you intend borrowing from any other source.

Information for the bank manager, and financial sources

Preliminary discussions can take place on the telephone and you must give a brief account of why you need an appointment. Prepare the proposition in plenty of time, sending any relevant documentation to the bank manager (or the manager of any other source of finance) prior to a meeting. This gives him plenty of time to consider your request.

The following information will be required:

1. A brief summary of the reason for the approach.
2. A short history and description of yourself, stating your age, education, professional qualifications, skills and specialisations. A prepared curriculum vitae is always helpful.
3. A list of personal means, for example, property, equipment, stocks and shares and any other asset that may be held for collateral against a loan.
4. The format of the practice, i.e. whether you are a single-handed practitioner or have a partner. The bank manager may want to know if your partner is using the same bank or obtaining a loan elsewhere.
5. Accounts, if you are buying an existing practice: these should be for the last three years if they are available; two years' accounts are the minimum you will need.
6. A detailed cash flow forecast and projected profit and loss account.
7. The maximum amount of finance you need to borrow. The finance must be negotiated precisely with fixed repayment details.
8. References of your character. These should be from people who have known you for a long time, who are not family or friends.

Once these details are finalised, one of the following methods of borrowing may be offered:

Overdrafts

An overdraft is the simplest and most convenient way of borrowing money. You may overdraw the account to an agreed limit. This method has the advantage of flexibility, but the interest rate may be very high. Since it will vary with the bank's base rate, it cannot be forecast accurately. This may prove very expensive if for any reason there is a sudden steep rise in the borrowing rates. The bank will ask for firm securities against the overdraft and it can withdraw the facility at its own discretion.

Bank loan

The bank will tailor the loan to meet your requirements. The loan is repaid at regular intervals. The disadvantage with a fixed interest loan is that if you have to borrow when interest rates are high, the interest on the loan will be fixed at a high rate. If the ordinary interest rates subsequently go down, the interest on the loan will not. Alternatively, if you borrow when the interest rates are low, and they then rise dramatically, you will have a relatively cheap loan.

Partnership capital

1. *Full partner*

If you are going into partnership, the partner will provide a percentage of the capital required for the practice. The most usual division is 50–50. This, of course, reduces the pressure on you to find the total capital, but it does mean the partner will recieve 50% of the profits. This active partner is known as a full partner. There are also two other options.

2. *Sleeping partners*

A sleeping partner is one who has put up capital in return for an eventual share in the profits, but does not take any part in running the practice.

3. *Salaried partners*

This type of partnership will give the partner a fixed salary regardless of the profit and loss of the practice. This may be preferable if you wish to keep the profits yourself, although you may agree to the partner receiving a small percentage of the profits.

The partner, therefore, may be active or sleeping, and it is a matter of luck and contacts if you find the person who is willing to risk money by backing your skills and talents. Partnership agreements are described later in the book, but it is important that both partners know and understand their financial obligations and rights.

Building societies

Building societies are a good source of money if you are buying property. However, they will not lend money for business expenditure.

Government money and grants

There are millions of pounds available for starting a new business and for expansion if you wish to ask for it. It is worth investigating what local and central government schemes or grants are available. You may only get help with rent and rates, but this is a start.

The bank manager or local authority, or the Manpower Services Commission may be helpful and the addresses can be found in the Appendix for the relevant government offices.

Finance and leasing companies

This source of money is becoming more widely used today. The companies offer a variety of schemes and it is important that you are clear what your obligations are under the leasing arrangement.

Many people choose to finance the purchase of equipment or a car by this method, since you do not have to pay the full cost at once.

The two most popular arrangements are:

1. *Finance leases or 'open ended' leases*

This type of lease supplies the money to make the purchase, the value of which at the end of the lease is known as the residual value. This value and any maintenance are the responsibility of the lessee.

Depreciation is estimated by subtracting the estimated residual value from the purchase price. You will pay the depreciation plus the interest during the period of the lease. At the end of the period agreed in the lease, the equipment or car is sold if it reaches more than the estimated residual value, and you will receive a refund. On the other hand, if it is sold at a loss, you will have to pay the difference.

2. *Contract hire or 'closed end' leases*

There are two types of scheme available—a non-maintenance and a full service leasing.
a. With non-maintenance leasing, the company provides everything except maintenance which remains the responsibility of the lessee.
b. In full service leasing, the company takes total responsibility for the equipment or car, including responsibility for any depreciation.
Under both these schemes it is possible to have replacements in case of an accident or fault.

3. *No deposit terms*

Under this scheme the finance company pays the supplier of the car or equipment and you enter into an agreement to repay the finance company interest over a fixed period. Ownership of the item then passes to you when the final payment has been made. This is a more expensive method, but there is often no requirement for security.

The choice will obviously depend on personal circumstances, the rates of interest charged by the companies and your tax position. If you own the equipment or car there will be tax allowances, but if you lease, the company will get the advantages.

KEEPING ACCOUNTS

Once you have raised the money, you must keep a careful record of all the financial transactions concerned with the practice. This is important, not only to check whether you are making a profit or loss, but also for the legal requirements involved in paying income tax.

Accounts may be kept in books, on cards, magnetic tapes or micro-film. Whichever method is used (and that is an individual choice for the practitioner), the accounts constitute the financial memory of the practice.

Name of the patient	Consultation/ treatment given	Fee charged £	Account sent	Account paid	Cheque £	Cash £
Mrs B. Rutherford	First examination	30.00	20.11.85	21.12.85	30.00	
Mr D. George	Injections	18.00	20.11.85	20.11.85		18.00
Miss V. Green	2nd Consultation and treatment	18.00	20.11.85	14.1.86	18.00	
	Total	66.00			48.00	18.00

Fig. 3.6 Diagram to show an example of the layout in a day book (see p. 58).

Date of receipt	Name of payer	Total	Cheque	Cash		Date	Payments	Cheque No.	Total
3.2.86	Mrs A. Jones	40.00	20.00	20.00		1.2.86	London Electricity	000001	98.65
						3.2.86	Rymans	000002	10.50
						4.2.86	G.P.O.	000003	160.00

Fig. 3.7 Layout of cash book or analysis ledger (see p. 58).

Often the practitioner is inexperienced at book-keeping, but you may be lucky and have a head for figures, or there may be a member of the staff who will help with the accounts.

Self-discipline

It cannot be stressed enough that you have to keep the books in order. It is largely a matter of self-discipline. Do it regularly and keep the books neat and tidy.

Light & heat	Rent & rates	Repairs & servicing	Telephone	Insurance	Laundry & cleaning	Petrol	Car repairs & servicing	Medical Supplies	Equipment	Printing & stationery	Accountancy & legal	Wages		Sundry
98.65										60.50				
			160.0											

Books of account

The tax inspector may wish to look at the books, and he will not be satisfied if he finds that you are not keeping proper records. It is unlikely that you will use either magnetic tapes or film in the first instance, so you will have to confine yourself to the more prosiac, but well-tested system of basic book-keeping to record and reconcile the accounts. The types of records you will be advised to keep by your accountant will depend on the size of the practice. When you start, you will require the following books:

The day book

This is sometimes called the fees book. In it, the income of the practice will be recorded on a daily basis, and you will be able to see who owes what at any given time. It shows whether you have been paid by cheque or in cash, which is recorded under the appropriate date, and it enables accounts to be sent out on a regular basis (see Fig 3.6). The total daily figure will correspond exactly with the receipts column in the cash book or analysis ledger.

The entries in the day book will also correlate with the appointments diary which may be viewed by the tax inspector if requested.

The cash book

This book provides an analysis and record of all the bank account receipts, money which has been received and the cheque payments made from the practice account. A typical cash book is shown in Figure 3.7.

The left hand side records the income. On the right hand side are the payments made for expenses, suitably analysed. It is necessary to have a heading for each column as it enables you to see at a glance the items and distribution of the expenses.

The number of each cheque you write must be recorded in sequence and lost or cancelled cheques must be noted.

Check the bank statements regularly when they arrive in conjunction with the cash book, so that you can note any standing orders or direct debit payments and obviate any errors.

The cash book, therefore, has to be checked with certain other items:

1. *Bank accounts*

The bank manager will recommend that you have two separate bank accounts, one for the practice expenditure which you will reconcile with the cash book, having numbered the cheques in sequence, and one for your personal needs. This is a necessity, as it does prevent any personal arrangements becoming confused with the practice finances.

2. *Bank statements*

Ask the bank to send these on a regular basis which can be

fortnightly or monthly. Check them carefully every time. They will show all the payments in and out of both the practice and personal accounts in separate statements. This will establish the balance in the bank and show any outstanding accounts.

3. *Invoices*

An invoice must be obtained, whenever possible, for any expenses related to the practice. These receipts must be filed in cheque number order. If they are petty cash expenses, they should be in date or numerical order, so that the accountant will be able to audit quickly at the end of the financial year.

The petty cash book and cash in the office

The petty cash book is used to record small items of expenditure, such as milk, tea, coffee or a taxi fare. Petty cash slips must be filled in, numbered, the receipts stapled to the slips and then filed numerically.

Petty cash must not come out of your pocket. It must be drawn by a regular cheque every week or month. You will cause confusion if you use cash which has been paid by a patient for petty cash purposes. It will be necessary to draw in the region of £30.00 to £50.00 according to the size of the practice. Have small notes and plenty of change. Do not keep large amounts of cash in the practice: it invites theft.

The cash can be kept in a locked cash box and it must be balanced every day.

Cash deposits

The cash received every day must ideally be banked daily. Time must be allowed for this. Try and have some cash in the practice for the patient who requires change from a banknote of a large denomination when paying his bill. Easy accessibility to a bank will save the embarrassment of having no change.

WAGES AND SALARIES SYSTEM

If you employ staff, you will have to record their gross pay, the National Insurance contributions and the tax deductions. Unless you have a very large staff, it is not worthwhile using a computerised system since it will not be cost effective and will be too complicated.

Instead, a manual system of paying wages is perfectly acceptable. You must use a system which is approved by the Inland Revenue, who provide forms which are quite adequate for wages records. There are also major stationers who produce wages books.

There are other financial rules and regulations to be complied with if you employ staff. Inform the local tax office that you are starting a wages system and they will arrange for tax tables to be sent to you. These will regularly be updated and it is possible to obtain advice from the tax office whenever it is necessary.

1. Pay As You Earn (PAYE)

As an employer, you are bound by law to deduct income tax from an employee's wages in accordance with the PAYE regulations, irrespective of whether the staff is employed full- or part-time. If you fail to deduct the tax you, and not the employee, will be liable for the tax. Income tax must be remitted to the Collector of Taxes by monthly instalments.

2. National Insurance contributions

These are deducted at the same time as PAYE and are remitted to the Collector of Taxes together with the employer's share of the National Insurance contribution.

3. Contracts of employment

Every employer is under an obligation to supply every employee who works more than sixteen hours each week, with a written statement of the conditions of employment. This must be supplied within thirteen weeks of the employment commencing. The terms which will be set out in the contract are described in Chapter 7.

TAXATION

In a book of this nature, it is not intended to deal with a subject as complicated as tax in any great detail. Taxation systems vary worldwide and your accountant will prepare the accounts and negotiate with the Inland Revenue on your behalf. He will know what you can and cannot claim against tax and the deadlines that have to be met for tax demands; he will also fill in the forms. Many of the communications from the Inland Revenue appear to be totally incomprehensible. When you receive anything from the Inland Revenue, send it on immediately to the accountant, as there are time limits for making appeals against assessments for tax and the submission of some documents, so do not delay in forwarding correspondence. Payment of tax is not something that can wait until after the profits are made, and delay in the payment of tax on the due date will result in interest being charged.

The tax year

The first accounts of the practice do not necessarily have to cover a period of twelve months and can be for a longer period. However, once the accounting date is chosen, this is then the date to which accounts have to be made up for subsequent years. Generally, the accountant will review the records after a year and will then advise on the optimum accounting date. Income tax assessments for a business which has been in existence for more than a year are generally issued in August or September with the tax becoming due in two equal instalments on the following 1st January and 1st July.

National Insurance contributions

In addition to the tax liability as a self-employed person, Class 4 National Insurance contributions have to be paid. These are collected together with the income tax. The contributions are calculated as a percentage of your net profit, subject to minimum or maximum levels of profit, which are varied each year by the government.

Similarly, you will be liable to pay Class 2 National Insurance contributions which are again at a rate fixed by the government each year. A card has to be obtained from your local Department of Health and Social Security office (DHSS) and a stamp obtained from the post office on a weekly basis. As an alternative, the contributions can be paid by direct debit by prior arrangement with the DHSS.

Tax and marriage

If a wife is earning an income for herself by working single handed and running a practice or carrying out some other freelance work, it is the husband who normally pays the tax due on her profits. He will claim a wife's earned income allowance as well as a married man's personal allowance.

A husband and wife can choose to have the wife's earned income taxed separately, but this is only an advantage for a couple who are in a high rate tax category. The application to be taxed separately has to be made jointly not earlier than six months and not later than twelve months after the relevant tax year. The wife's earnings will continue to be taxed separately until a joint notice of withdrawal is given.

Principal allowable business expenses

Certain expenses you incur in the course of your work can be deducted from your income, but they must be 'wholly and exclusively incurred in your profession'. This will then give the amount of your income which is liable for tax once these expenses have been deducted. Claim everything to which you are entitled and be guided by the accountant.

The following list will give you a guide:
1. The running costs of the premises including rent and rates, heating and lighting, and any repairs and renewals.
2. Medical and office equipment.
3. Uniform, professional clothing, laundry and cleaning.
4. Printing, postage and stationery.
5. Wages and salaries to employees, together with National Insurance contributions.
6. Professional subscriptions, and medical periodicals and journals.
7. Travelling and attendances at post-registration courses and conferences.
8. Legal fees.
9. Insurance.
10. Accountancy fees.
11. Hiring and leasing charges.
12. Entertaining staff, for example, giving a Christmas party.
13. Bad debts.
14. Running expenses of a car, excluding such proportion which is attributable to private use.

Home as a practice. If you are using part of your home as a surgery or practice, a certain proportion of the running costs of the house can be claimed as a business expense. This can be as high as two-thirds, providing you can convince the tax inspector that this is the proportion used 'wholly and exclusively' for the practice. Your accountant may advise against this procedure, as if you wish to sell the property in the future, capital gains tax will have to be paid; thus any tax advantages are lost. Capital gains tax will only apply to an owner-occupied house, not a rented one.

Depreciation. This is the method by which capital expenditure items, such as the car, medical equipment and permanent fixtures and fittings, are written off over their working life. It is a record allowing allocation of some of the cost of the asset to be spread over the appropriate time period. This period will be determined by how long the working life of the asset is likely to be.

Advice from the accountant will be invaluable here, especially when you are calculating the depreciation of equipment and a car.

Stock valuation

If you are holding any stock at the end of the financial year, it has to be valued for tax purposes. It is advisable to have a monthly and annual inventory of stock to enable you to keep a tight control on your budget and spending, and, therefore, have control of the valuation when it is time to prepare the annual accounts. The Inland Revenue will pay close attention to the manner in which businesses value their stock, so take advice about the basis of valuing stock. It will obviously make a difference to the profits if closing stock is valued on a different basis from the opening stock and vice versa.

Value Added Tax (VAT)

At present the services offered by registered health professionals are not chargeable under the VAT system. Therefore, the practice will not be registered for VAT purposes (see The Value Added Tax Act 1983 Group 7). The arduous task of filling in more forms and records is, therefore, avoided. This does mean, however, that as you cannot charge VAT so you cannot claim VAT charged to you on any accounts payable by the practice, for example, telephone charges, printing, or building works. Allow for this in the costing.

Pensions and retirement

It may seem a little premature to discuss retirement when you are first starting in private practice, but it is an area which is sometimes overlooked.

Employed people can enjoy pension benefit schemes as part of their employment package, but when you become self-employed there is not the same degree of security. You will have to make arrangements for a pension and provision for your family and dependants, and for any other responsibilities. This is discussed more fully in the next chapter.

The State pension will not be adequate enough to provide you with a comfortable and secure retirement. Therefore, it is possible to pay premiums into a personal pension policy from the outset. The tax legislation relating to the allowability of premiums is complex, but at present you can pay 17.5% of your net profit into a pension fund or funds. Choose a flexible policy which has a low basic annual premium with an option to top up in the good financial years and reduce or waive entirely in the years of low profit. The accountant will advise you on how much top up premium to pay prior to the end of the financial year. It must be remembered that old policies cannot be encashed prior to the retirement date without incurring a heavy penalty.

As insurance is such a wide and complex field, it is advisable to obtain the advice of a reputable broker as soon as possible. Insurance is discussed in the next chapter.

Investment advice

If the practice expands in the future, it may be necessary to use the services of a stockbroker.

The stock market has a history of good investment by its brokers, but there will be dips and troughs. If you are sensible about what you buy and sell, it can enhance your long-term capital growth. Some brokers advise unit trusts as a more reliable source of investment, although it is not practical to invest less than £1000 since the spread of the portfolio of the trust is usually very wide.

If you make a lot of money and you decide to seek an alternative to stocks and shares, then maybe an investment in Lloyds of London is the step to take.

Reminder note

The business of investing and lending money is extremely diverse and dynamic, so look around carefully. Your professional services are free until they are paid for, that is, the accounts receivable only materialise into cash when the patient eventually settles the account. If patients delay payment, then the interest lost can be considerable. It becomes expensive and embarrassing. If there is a cash crisis, do discuss it with your financial advisers. They are there to help you.

PRACTITIONER CHECK LIST

1. Have you set out a plan in writing?
2. Is your potential profit worth the effort you will put in?
3. Do you know how much capital you require?
4. From what source are you going to seek capital?
5. Are there any bad debts if you are considering buying an established practice?
6. What are your securities?
7. Have you drawn up a cash flow forecast and a profit and loss budget?
8. Is your present bank one you can use or is it too small to have the necessary funds?
9. Have you organised two separate accounts?
10. Have you costed your own time properly and established a fee structure in line with other practices?
11. Have you established all the legal charges?
12. Have you discussed your tax position with the accountant?

4

Legal implications and insurance

Do as you would be done by.
Charles Kingsley 1819–1875

ETHICS

Ethics is the branch of philosophy concerned with human character and conduct. For the medical practitioner, ethics are the principles of conduct governing the profession to which he belongs, which oblige its members to conform to accepted standards of conduct. Many of the principles can be identified and articulated into a reasonably straightforward and easily understandable set of rules which establish quite clearly what is acceptable professional behaviour and what is not.

The present century has seen major changes in moral attitudes, rapid developments in medical and surgical techniques, and a relentless advance in technology, all of which have created particular ethical dilemmas for medical practitioners. Although many of the problems have been resolved, a consensus has not been reached on all of them.

Rules of professional conduct

The ethical principles which are regarded as fundamental to the practice of medicine are embodied in the professional and ethical rules of conduct pertinent to each of the health care professions, and it is very important that every practitioner is familiar with them. It is only by strict adherence to ethical conduct that patients may continue to receive not only the highest standards of clinical care, but also correct professional behaviour. Any practitioner faced with a situation for which there appear to be no obvious guidelines must seek immediate help and advice from his professional organisation.

MEDICAL PRACTITIONERS AND THE LAW

There is a close relationship between ethical and legal responsibilities and many occasions where ethical practice and the 'legal standard of care' are inseparable. 'The legal standard of care' may be expressed as the duty to exercise reasonable care and skill.

The contract with the patient

Prior to the National Health Service Act 1946, medical law in England was largely dominated by the contractual relationship between doctor and patient. The services of the practitioner were provided under direct contract with the patient, and the law which developed around medicine was derived from the law of contract.

The present position for those practising privately, is that advice or treatment is given in pursuance of a contract between the practitioner and the patient which commits the practitioner to exercise skill and care in the treatment undertaken. There is, in addition, a common law duty of care which binds any practitioner who undertakes treatment of a patient to exercise the legal standard of care irrespective of a contract between them. The failure to do so, may give rise to an action in what is known legally as tort of negligence.

Breach of contract

Additionally, failure to exercise skill and care may give rise to an action for breach of contract. In general, however, the existence of the contract, in private practice, does not affect the legal obligations of the practitioner. It is important to understand that a medical practitioner's duty of care arises quite independently of a contract with the patient. It is based quite simply on the fact that treatment has been undertaken. It applies to treatment given gratuitously, in an emergency or at the scene of a road accident. Once a practitioner has taken it upon himself to treat the patient in whatever the circumstances, he is bound by law to exercise appropriate skill and care. The liability arising from improper performance of that skill is not therefore based on the law of contract, but on the general principles of the law of negligence.

A further example of the principle that the liability arises independently of a contract is found where payment is to be made for the practitioner's services by a person other than the patient. It is a principle of English law that none but the parties to a contract may sue for breach of it, but it is firmly established that the patient who suffers harm may sue the practitioner for negligence notwithstanding the fact that the practitioner was retained and was to be paid by another person. Therefore, a medical practitioner who undertakes the treatment of a patient gratuitously, or for a payment made by the patient or by a third party or in any circumstances whatsoever, owes the patient a legal duty of care, and a breach of that duty may give rise to an action by the patient for negligence.

Negligence

It is impossible to identify all the conceivable instances of medical negligence or to state whether an act or omission or course of conduct will or will not give rise to an allegation of negligence. Some examples may be: failure to attend a patient, failure to refer a patient when appropriate, failure to use all available diagnostic aids, failure to disclose relevant clinical information to another practitioner who is treating a patient, failure to use X-ray facilities if required or to send samples for analysis.

A patient who is injured physically or psychologically by the negligence of a practitioner may sue for and recover damages. The dividing line between an error of judgement and negligence can be difficult to draw.

If a patient claims damages for alleged negligence, and the claim is denied, the matter can then be made the subject of an action in the County Court or the High Court, depending on the level of damages anticipated. The matter is decided by a judge who will hear the case for both sides. Witnesses will be called and the patient's case notes may be examined. If appropriate, damages will be awarded. They may be awarded for pain, suffering, incapacity, the necessity for further treatment and/or loss of earnings. If there is a continuing result from the negligence, they may also be awarded for future pain and loss of earnings. The general rule is, that in order to recover damages for personal injury, the action must be started within three years of the date on which the patient became aware that a particular treatment could be the cause of the problem giving rise to the claim. If action is not started within that time, then the practitioner may have a defence based on the statute of limitations, irrespective of the merit of the claim.

It cannot be over-emphasised that not all mishaps will be ascribed to negligence. It will be for the judge to decide whether in a case of alleged negligence the practitioner has, in fact, been negligent. The guiding rule is for the practitioner to stay within his level of competence and skill, and to take every care that he applies his professional training and expertise properly.

Standard of care

What is the legal standard of care and skill required of the practitioner? In the general law of negligence, the standard of 'the reasonable man' applies, but where a person represents that he has a special skill or knowledge, the law demands standards appropriate to that. The medical practitioner will therefore be liable in an action for negligence if he fails to exercise that degree of care and skill expected of the average practitioner of the profession to which he belongs. He will not be judged by the standard of the least competent, nor by the standard of the most highly competent, but by the standard of the ordinarily careful and competent practitioner. The standard of skill is also related to the status and experience of the practitioner.

For example, less will be expected of a junior house surgeon than of a senior consultant with many years' experience. Circumstances are also relevant. It would not be reasonable to expect the same degree of care to apply to treatment given to a victim of a major train disaster in circumstances which are very difficult and where there are few facilities, as to that given in well-equipped surroundings in ideal conditions.

Nevertheless, the care and skill must be acceptable, given those circumstances. Treatment does not have to be perfect, but liability may arise if the practitioner fails to take the care he ought to have taken or to use the skills he ought to have used at the time.

Consent

a. *Adults*

No adult patient can be forced to have treatment without giving consent, the only exception being certain groups of patients who come within the Mental Health Act 1983. If, therefore, treatment is given without consent, the patient may be able to sue for unlawful assault, which is an offence under the Offence Against the Persons Act 1861, Section 47.

Consent is not often explicitly stated in words or written down when the patient initially seeks help from a practitioner. There is an implied consent to examination, treatment investigations, and tests. There are times when explicit consent is required, for example, before a surgical operation or an investigation or test when a general anaesthetic is given, and a patient will be asked to sign a consent form. To be effective, consent must be what is called 'informed consent'. It must be given freely and willingly, after the nature and purpose of the treatment or investigatory procedure has been clearly explained by a qualified practitioner. It is important that the patient understands what is going to happen to him, and, therefore, the person obtaining the consent must ensure that the matter is discussed without the use of complicated medical terms more than is necessary. If inadequate or misleading explanations are given, the apparent consent given by the patient may be considered ineffective. It is not necessary, however, to tell the patient of every conceivable misfortune which could occur; the principal objective is to ensure that sufficient information is given to enable him to make a reasonable decision regarding the consent which he is being asked to give. It is a question of professional judgement in deciding what you must or must not tell the patient. It is a matter of courtesy, in any case, to explain what you are going to do, what effect it may have or any side-effects which may result.

It is worth noting here that patients are very vulnerable. They may be in pain, anxious or nervous. What may seem quite routine and ordinary to the practitioner may be very worrying and rather frightening to the patient. Although you may have explained a procedure many many times, do not be casual about it, it will be the first time your patient has heard it. He is entitled to a proper explanation.

b. *Minors*

Parliament has laid down that consent to medical treatment can be given at the age of 16 years in the United Kingdom. Under this age, consent of the parent is normally requested. This does not mean that the child's consent is not also required, but there is no specified age below which a child can be treated whether he likes it or not. Generally speaking, the older the child, the more his wishes must be respected.

Confidentiality

This is a very difficult area. In general, doctors are not allowed to pass on to a third party information they have acquired in a professional capacity about a patient. This general principle is regarded as a cornerstone of the doctor/patient relationship. It has been accepted, and is followed by practitioners in the other health professions. However, many inroads have been made into it. Some have been made by the law, for example, doctors have to notify the local Health Authority of certain infectious diseases. To prevent the spread of these conditions, most people would regard the disclosure of such information as totally acceptable. Another exception may arise in the case of a patient whose condition makes him a danger to the community. Such cases are fortunately rare, and the disclosure of such information may be essential for the well-being not only of the patient, but of others.

There are circumstances when duty as a citizen over-rules duty to one's patient. Thus, confidentiality may be overborn by the law or outweighed by a wider obligation to the community in general. Despite these exceptions, the principle is that professional confidences may not be revealed to anyone without the patient's consent.

When a patient is referred from one practitioner to another, there is implied consent by the patient for information relating to his medical condition to be disclosed. It would be detrimental to the patient if the referring practitioner failed to pass on relevant clinical information. There is, fortunately, a high degree of respect for notes, records and clinical information by all members of the medical professions. Without it the referral system would hardly function. It goes without saying that information received from a referring practitioner is treated with the same confidence as if it had been given directly by the patient. A practitioner who is asked for confidential information by anybody other than a health care professional, can avoid problems if he obtains the patient's consent to the disclosure. This is normally willingly and freely given, but if it is not, there must be a very important reason for the practitioner not to respect the patient's wishes. What can the patient do if information is disclosed without his consent? The situation arises very rarely, and he can sue for breach of confidence.

Breach of confidentiality

In a court of law, a practitioner can be compelled by a judge or any competent legal authority to disclose information. This has been summarised by Lord Denning when he was Master of the Rolls:

The only profession which I know which is given a privilege from disclosing information to a court of law is the legal profession, and then it is not the privilege of the lawyer, but of his client. Take the clergyman, the banker, or the medical man. None of these is entitled to refuse to answer when directed to by a judge. Let me not be mistaken. The judge will respect the confidences which each member of these honourable professions receives in the course of it, and will not direct him to answer unless not only it is relevant, but also a proper and, indeed, necessary question in the course of justice to be put and answered. A judge is the person entrusted on behalf of the community, to weigh these conflicting interests.

Minors

A person aged 16 or over can usually expect compliance with the wish that his or her parents must not be told that he has sought advice or treatment.

A very young person or child usually presents no problems. He is unlikely to seek medical help, independently, so reference can be made to his parents. However, difficulties may arise when dealing with young patients in the 14–16 year-old age group. In general, a very strong case would have to be made for totally ignoring the wishes of this group. Therefore, it is advisable to try and persuade the young person to involve his parents.

Vicarious liability

As we have seen, a medical practitioner is obliged to exercise the legal standard of care at all times when personally treating a patient. In addition to personal responsibility for the application of a proper standard of care, the practitioner may also be responsible for the acts or omissions of personnel employed in the practice whether they are professional or non-professional. This obligation is called vicarious liability and arises from the legal relationship of master and servant, although this is nowadays called, more appropriately, the employer–employee relationship.

It is a well-established principle of English law that where a servant (employee) commits a tort (an action for which damages may be sought, i.e. negligence) in the course of employment, the employer is vicariously liable for the consequences of that act. For example, if a van driver negligently knocks down and injures a pedestrian, the pedestrian is able to hold the van driver's employer liable. The van driver is also liable, but there is a distinction between the nature of the driver's liability and that of the employer.

The driver is liable as he is responsible for knocking over the pedestrian and personally owes him a duty of care which he failed to exercise. The employer owes no personal duty of care to the pedestrian but his liability is imposed on him because he is the employer and the act was committed by his employee during the course of his employment.

A practitioner is vicariously liable for the acts or omissions of his employees to whom he delegates responsibility for treatment. The practitioner must be completely satisfied that the person to whom he has delegated responsibility is competent and capable of carrying out the treatment in a professional manner. It is important that the degree of skill, experience and knowledge required for the treatment is not beyond that of the person asked to undertake it. If an action for alleged negligence should arise, the employee will be personally liable and the practitioner vicariously liable.

Another situation which can arise is where a professional person works in a practice and treats patients, but is not an employee of the practitioner, i.e. he is a self-employed locum or another private practitioner; people who work in this way are called independent contractors. It is clear that the employer–employee relationship does not exist in these circumstances, but the practitioner has 'employed' another professional to undertake the treatment of patients in his practice.

The general rule is that an employer is not liable for the acts of an independent contractor, but there are circumstances where, due to the special nature of the work, the employer himself owes a legal duty of care which he cannot delegate to others and this situation applies in medical practice. Thus the practitioner is liable for the acts or omissions of another professional even though that person is not an employee of the practitioner. It has been said that 'if an employer is under a duty to a person or class of persons he is liable if that duty is not performed and damage thereby results, and cannot evade that liability by delegating the performance of that duty to an independent contractor' (Salmond on Torts).

Therefore the practitioner has a liability for the acts or omissions of those working in or for the practice irrespective of employment status.

Chaperones

Experience and good judgement will tell you when a chaperone is needed for a consultation. Since some medical examinations and treatments are of a very personal nature, care must be taken to ensure that a chaperone is present, where appropriate, so that neither the practitioner nor the patient is compromised. If in doubt, ask for one to be present.

Chaperones must be as discreet and unobtrusive as possible, and can be any member of staff. They must maintain and respect the confidentiality of the patient at all times. If the patient will not consent to a chaperone being present, then you can refuse to treat him.

Drugs and injections

Drugs and injections must be administered properly and kept under lock and key at all times. The patient must know what he is being given and if there are any side-effects. He may be over-sensitive or allergic to certain products. Correct advice must always be given to the patient.

PROFESSIONAL CONDUCT

In addition to being subject to the Civil and Criminal law, the practitioner must abide by the professional rules of conduct relevant to his particular profession. The medical professions regulate their own codes of conduct and administer disciplinary sanctions against their members who breach them. Modern society, changing professional relationships and roles and the development of new techniques and treatment make it almost impossible for any professional group to tightly define the parameters of accepted practice. Codes of conduct, therefore, increasingly stress the importance of the integrity and personal judgement of individual practitioners to act always in the best interests of the patient. A thorough knowledge of the professional rules is strongly recommended.

Disciplinary procedures

All professional organisations have disciplinary powers for dealing with registered practitioners who have either been convicted of an offence by a court, even if the offence did not involve professional misconduct, or been involved in an allegation of serious professional misconduct. Complaints may come from colleagues or members of the public, and the precise investigatory procedures

and sanctions which may be applied vary from profession to profession. The areas of professional conduct most likely to give rise to disciplinary procedures are:
1. Neglect or disregard of professional responsibilities to patients.
2. Abuse of professional privileges or skills.
3. Conduct detrimental to the reputation of the profession.
4. Advertising, canvassing or related offences.
A practitioner asked to appear at an investigation conducted by his professional organisation may be legally represented. It is strongly advised that practitioners familiarise themselves with the rules of conduct relevant to their particular profession.

Complaints from a patient

These usually relate to fees, practice management or clinical treatment:

1. *Fees*

Fees must be in line with those charged by other practitioners in the area. Excessive charges are extremely unprofessional. You may have spent a great deal of time and effort on a particular patient and it is proper for you to charge for that, but you must be prepared and able to justify your account to the patient. He is paying for it, either from his own resources or through his medical insurance premiums.

Occasionally, the patient does not improve as a result of your treatment, and may feel aggrieved when asked to pay the bill. This is a very unsatisfactory situation. No practitioner can guarantee a cure, relief, remission or even alleviation of the patient's problem. There are many conditions which prove very resistant to treatment and an unhappy dissatisfied patient is very difficult to deal with. Professionally, it is your responsibility to do your best, or refer the patient to somebody else if your treatment has not succeeded.

2. *Clinical treatment*

Complaints in respect of clinical treatment may range from those of a very trivial nature, to those which are serious. In general, most complaints can be dealt with by the practitioner using common sense and tact. In serious cases of alleged clinical mispractice the practitioner should contact his professional organisation immediately for help and advice. Do not be tempted to deal with this yourself. There may be an eventual court case, and any action taken without appropriate advice could be very damaging.

KEEPING MEDICAL RECORDS

If there is disciplinary action or court proceedings take place, medical records are vital for reference and will generally have to be disclosed (The Administration of Justice Act 1970).

If you are approached by solicitors, the public health authority or the police for access to your records, you must obtain advice from the professional organisation to which you belong before any disclosures are made.

It is, therefore, absolutely essential to keep accurate, comprehensive, concise and up-to-date legible patients' records. They should include dates of attendance, diagnosis, details of treatment and drugs, copies of all letters relevant to the patient and the date of discharge. They must be stored safely and access to them must be restricted to as few people as possible to preserve confidentiality. Make sure notes are not left where they may be read by other patients or unauthorised persons.

Medical records can be stored in a computer. This should not present any difficulty either in terms of access or in preserving confidentiality, but you will have to comply with the requirements of the Data Protection Act 1984. At present, it is necessary to keep handwritten or typed copies of all clinical information stored in a computer. Records must be kept for a minimum period of eight years. In the case of children they must be retained until the child reaches 25 years of age.

The appointment book

This book is a daily record of the patient's attendance, and the contract you have made with the patient.

If it is requested, it may have to be produced in a court of law or at a disciplinary hearing. The book must be kept carefully with clear and legible handwriting.

ADVERTISING

The Medical Act 1858 stated that the purpose of establishing the Medical Register was to enable 'persons requiring medical aid to distinguish qualified from unqualified practitioners'. Subsequently, the dissemination of information has been and continues to be a controversial area and the subject of much debate. Practitioners are often unsure how to make the existence of their practices known without infringing the rules of professional conduct on advertising.

At the present time, you may not directly or indirectly canvass, appeal, solicit or tout for patients. You must not, therefore, print a letter announcing your practice and distribute it indiscriminately. You may not advertise on the radio, on television or in the national press. There are, however, several quite acceptable ways of announcing the availability of your practice and initiating public relations in the community.

Choosing a name or title for the practice

1. It is usual to use your own name and have it on the front door and on the practice writing paper. For example: Mr D. French FRCS, or Mrs D. Barnes MCSP. In addition to the designatory letters, you may state your profession. This makes it clear to a patient what you actually practise as he may not be familiar with qualification abbreviations or what they mean.

2. You may practise under a collective name, i.e. The West Cliffe Clinic, and in certain professions you may also state the specialisation of the practice, for example The West Cliffe Sports Injuries Clinic.

Professional door-plates

Lettering on door-plates must be confined to the name and qualifications of the practitioner and the hours the practice is open. If there is more than one practitioner in the building, the name-plates must be of similar size and form so that the attention of the patient is not drawn to one rather than another.

Announcing the opening of the practice

1. *Writing letters*

It is quite proper for you to notify other medical practitioners that you are in practice. The announcement must be addressed to the practitioner personally, be brief, informed and contain qualifications, any specialist skills and the location of the practice. A letter may also be sent if you change your address. All communications must be sent in a sealed envelope. Advice as to whether it is ethical for you to contact local clubs, interest groups, health studios or commercial gymnasia should be sought from your professional organisation.

2. *Telephone directories and yellow pages*

At the time of writing, the general principle for entries in telephone directories or Yellow Page directories is that the insertion should be informatory only. It must not draw attention to the individual practitioner by the use of bold or large type. No reference should be made to qualifications not relevant to the practice. It is customary for practitioners in the same area and from the same profession to take a block booking in the Yellow Pages. This is acceptable providing the list does not place any of the participants at a disadvantage (see Fig. 4.1).

3. *The local press*

Certain professions permit the insertion of an announcement in the local paper. It must be factual, restrained and concise, stating the name and qualifications of the practitioner, the location and telephone number. No other information should be included.

Sale of goods

If you are responsible for helping in the design of some apparatus, equipment or any other medical preparation, you must refrain from being associated with the commercial and financial aspects of the product. Your name must not appear in any advertisement for the goods. You must not sell, endorse or promote the sale of goods, if by doing so you gain an unfair professional advantage over other practitioners. The practice premises must not be used for the sale of goods to patients unless they are necessary for treatment, for example, a dispensary attached to a surgery. Any interest in a commercial venture must not be used to promote or advance your professional practice.

Publicity and the media

The growing interest in medical matters and the media coverage this has generated, may place a practitioner in difficulties if he is

```
CHARTERED AND
STATE REGISTERED
PHYSIOTHERAPISTS

James D. West MCSP SRP
2 Station Road, Turville.
Turville 467321 and 789614

V. Morgan MCSP SRP
Shrubland House,
Turville Heath.
Turville 246819

P. Jenkins MCSP SRP
41 Virginia Grove, Turville.
Turville 621344

B. B. Downside MCSP SRP
The Vale,
606 Avenue Road, Turville.
Turville 881243 and 881779


The above Private Practitioners are
registered under the Professions
Supplementary to Medicine Act 1960.
```

Fig. 4.1 Example of a Yellow Pages insertion.

asked to comment or advise publicly. There is nothing improper in taking part in radio and television debates or agreeing to interviews in the national or local press provided attention is not drawn either to the location of the practice or to any special skills or qualifications held by the practitioner other than those which identify his ability to speak with confidence and authority on a particular topic. Self-laudatory or promotional comments must be avoided. Advice and information should be strictly professional and accurate. No correspondence must be entered into as a result of any publicity gained through the media.

INSURANCE

Insurance is both compulsory and voluntary, since you will have to pay compulsory National Insurance contributions. You must protect yourself, however, against the financial consequences of an accident or unfortunate events, which may occur in both professional and private life, by making provision for adequate insurance cover. This is a voluntary insurance, but extremely necessary whatever your age for the reasons that have already been described. The suitability of the insurance policies you will wish to take out will be based on initial discussions with your accountant and then the insurance broker, and they must be designed to fulfil your needs and cover all potential risks. Insurance may also be available through your professional organisation, so it is worth checking this source.

The contract with the insurance company

Insurance contracts are known as contracts of *Uberrimae Fidei* (of the utmost good faith) between the person buying the protection, that is, the policy holder and the insurance company. There is a heavy duty on the person purchasing the protection to disclose all material facts. Incorrect, incomplete or misleading information will invalidate the policy. Insurance is expensive so seek the advice of the broker to find the right terms to cover any risks and suit your particular requirements. The consideration of the insurance company will be the premium you pay.

The following insurances will be necessary:

1. Surgery or practice insurance

Many of the large companies now offer a comprehensive policy especially designed for medical practices. The cover provided will include:

a. *Contents*

Accidental loss, destruction or damage to contents. When estimating the value of the contents make sure you include furniture, fixtures and fittings, books, linens, stationery, carpets, curtains, files and filing systems, equipment and drugs. If a fire destroys the building all these items will have to be replaced at current prices so make sure you know how much it would cost to buy them. The companies often send a check list so you can be sure you have not forgotten anything, and it is wise to regularly update the insurance.

b. *Building insurance*

If you own or are responsible for insuring the building, insurance can be taken out to cover accidental loss, destruction or damage. If you practise from home, the building will probably be covered by the householder's existing policy and this can be extended to include the practice and its contents.

c. *Consequential loss*

This insurance is taken out against loss of earnings if the premises are so badly damaged you are unable to practise while repairs and renovations are being assessed and carried out. It is a very useful protection as most people have financial commitments which have to be met even if there is no income. Also staff will have to be paid until the practice is functioning again.

2. Legal liability insurance

Never admit liability. Make sure you have the appropriate insurance and if there is an accident or injury, fill in the necessary forms and send them to the insurers immediately. They will then hand them straight on to the underwriters. The main liability insurances are:

a. *Professional liability insurance*

The payment of a full annual subscription to the professional organisation or Society provides cover for liability if the patient receives damage or injury in the course of treatment. This is usual in most countries; see addresses for reference in Appendix 0. However, in some cases this is inadequate as legal cases have now been recorded where the damages awarded to the patient plus the litigation costs have exceeded the cover carried by the professional organisation. The practitioner must seek additional cover to meet the individual needs.

b. *Public liability insurance*

This insurance is essential. It covers a member of the public who has an accident on your premises, unconnected with the treatment.

For example, a patient may fall because of faulty or badly fitted carpeting, and sustain a fractured ankle. This is a serious injury and at the very least may prevent the patient from leading a normal life for some time, or at worst prevent him from working and earning a living. He will seek compensation from you. He will not have a claim, however, if the carpet is in perfectly good order and he fell because he did not look where he was going. If you are leasing or renting premises, make sure carpets in any part of the building likely to be used by patients are insured either by you or the landlord. The patient will also have a claim against you, providing he asked you to look after his valuables, for such items as jewellery or clothing, whilst on the premises.

c. *Employers' liability insurance*

This is a compulsory insurance covering both permanent and temporary staff against claims made for death or injury incurred by an employee whilst working in your practice. Cover will also include damages awarded against you and any legal costs which may be incurred if you defend an action. The premium is usually based at a rate percentage of the total salaries bill. The appropriate certificate must be visibly displayed in the practice as evidence that the insurance has been obtained.

3. Car insurance

This is obviously essential. If you are intending to use the car for visiting patients at home or in a hospital, clinic or nursing home, the insurance company must be informed. If the car is already insured for personal use, then the cover will have to be extended to include business use. If you have an accident and it can be shown that the car was being used for purposes for which it is not covered, the insurance company will not accept liability for the claim. This may be extremely high, especially if the accident is a serious one and the car or third party suffers substantial damage. If the claim is rejected, you will also have to pay for the other party's damage if the accident was your fault. If you should lose your driving licence, it is possible to insure for hiring transport.

4. Personal accident insurance

If you are the sole contributor to the family income, it is worth taking out this policy in case of death or an accident causing temporary total disablement. This policy is sometimes linked to a life assurance cover and a pension.

5. Permanent health insurance

If an illness is prolonged or there is permanent long-term disability, this insurance is designed to cover the incapacity of the practitioner. Incapacity to work means the total inability of the insured, by reason of sickness or injury, to follow his occupation. The premiums are payable at a choice of intervals and the broker will advise you on which method is the most beneficial. You may be required to take a medical examination by the insurance company's doctor to establish or confirm the disability. There are certain exclusions, such as the excessive use of drugs or alcohol, and pregnancy or childbirth. If at a later date you return to work on a part-time basis, then a reduced payment will be made related to your previous earnings. The insurance company will check with the accountant the previous three years of figures of the practice before making any payment on a permanent basis.

6. Private medical insurance

This is entirely different from the permanent health insurance. It is a matter of personal choice if you decide to take out one of the large company schemes. The premiums can be fairly high, but it does mean that if you require immediate medical attention then you can take advantage of the services of the private sector without worrying too much about the size of other medical colleagues' accounts!

7. Drugs

Inform the insurance company if you carry drugs in the car, and also if they are in the practice.

8. Money

You can obtain cover for the loss of money in the practice, such as cash, credit cards, stamps etc. As the practice expands, so will the amount of money which you have to deal with every day. The insurers will expect certain precautions to be taken before they will insure the money, so even if you do not take out the insurance, the premium on the property may be higher as there is more likelihood of theft and burglary. It is wise to avoid the same regular route if you carry a large amount of money.

9. Mortgage minder

If you are ill for a long period or suffer a serious accident, there is a policy which can be taken out to pay monthly mortgage repayments, so you do not lose your home or practice. This policy will also pay off the mortgage in full if you become permanently disabled and cannot return to work again.

10. Life policies

There is no fixed amount for you to aim at when deciding how much life assurance you may need. If you are married, decide what income the surviving partner might require, calculate your outstanding commitments if you should die prematurely and choose a policy which will be flexible for your requirements. Make sure the contract and any surrender terms involved in the policy are explained to you. The accountant will give advice on how much of your income can be committed on a regular and long-term basis. Review the terms regularly and then you will not lose money.

There are several kinds of policies: the endowment-with-profits policies are the most popular. They can be expensive, but they provide a means of protecting dependants in the event of death and provide for a comfortable retirement. Premiums are paid for a fixed number of years, and if you live to the end of the period you receive the sum assured. If you die while you are still making payments, then the money will pass to your family or heirs. These policies are often linked to mortgage repayments.

You will get the largest cover for the least outlay with a term assurance policy. You may have an option in it to change it later into a more valuable policy, so it may become a convertible term policy. Term assurance is when the premiums are paid for a fixed number of years, usually not less than ten, and then if you die, the sum assured will be paid out. If you survive until the term has ended, then the policy pays out nothing.

SEEKING LEGAL ADVICE

At the beginning of this book, the importance of using a solicitor was emphasised. A professional medical practice is not routine work for a solicitor, and no two solicitors' practices are the same. Some are much more experienced in this area, so a systematic approach is probably the best way of finding a solicitor. There are a number of occasions when you will need legal advice.

The courts

If you are sued by a patient for professional reasons, initially you will contact your professional organisation and be guided by them. However, you will need legal representation if the case comes to court or if there is a disciplinary hearing by the professional body. The professional liability insurance policy will cover the costs of the hearing and so it is wise to have legal advice from a solicitor.

A partnership agreement

If two or more persons agree to carry on a business with a view to making a profit, then they form a partnership, whether it is formalised by a legal agreement or not. Each partner is individually responsible for the liabilities and debts of the practice as a whole, so if one absconds with all the money, the one left behind is responsible for the debts. Therefore, it is advisable and sensible to ask a solicitor to draw up an agreement, which will provide a guarantee. On the other hand, it does not necessarily mean that if you share the profits, you have to have a partnership. You may pay your staff on a profit-sharing or bonus scheme, but they need not be partners.

Someone in your family may lend you money for the practice; you will then pay him interest on the loan and the capital will be repaid on an agreed basis. In order to clarify that the relative is neither a partner nor involved in the day-to-day running of the practice, it is wise to have a simple agreement relating to the loan drawn up by a solicitor.

You will, therefore, have to decide what form of partnership you want. The following points should be considered when an agreement is drawn up:

a. How are the profits to be shared, equally or not?

b. How are the losses to be apportioned?
c. Are the profits to be distributed according to the work done, i.e. the number of hours worked, or the number of patients seen?
d. The amount of salary to be drawn by each partner must be specified, whether it is a sum or a percentage.
e. What expenses can be charged by each partner against the practice?
f. Time off and holiday periods must be agreed between the partners.
g. If one partner leaves the practice, an agreement must be drawn up restricting him from practising within a certain radius of the practice for a specified time. The restriction has to be reasonable for both parties in that it protects the interests of the practice, but it does not place an unacceptable restraint on the departing partner.

Written agreements, minutes and agendas are essential if the partnership is to be successful, otherwise discussions, decisions or policies will be forgotten, delayed or abandoned.

Duration of a partnership

The agreement drafted by the solicitor must have a starting date and a date of termination, since although partnerships always start off on a sunny note, it is an unfortunate fact of life that relationships do not always remain in this happy state. The time limit of the termination date must specify a period of notice to be given in the event of the partnership breaking up, if three, five or ten years is unacceptable.

Admitting or expelling a partner

Each partner has to consent to changes in an agreement, but it is a wise idea to include a facility in the agreement for admitting a new partner and expelling one if necessary. No agreement can foresee what might happen to a partnership—like marriage it involves a good deal of give and take. If it reaches a point where bad relationships are affecting the practice, the patients will certainly be aware of them, so the necessary action will have to be taken before things get worse. Compulsory retirement is better than expulsion.

A limited company

This can be a useful tool if you employ staff, and for administrative and medical supply purposes. The solicitor will clarify the tax advantages for you and the company will be an offshoot of the practice, with yourself as a director, excluding your professional qualifications since this could limit your liability within your professional scope. Always seek advice from the professional organisation as well as the solicitor if there is any hint of commercialism.

The police

If for any reason to do with the practice and its patients, you have the unpleasant or embarrassing position of being involved with the police, in order to prevent any ill will, contact a solicitor immediately and your professional organisation.

Conveyancing

Buying an established practice and the searches that will have to be carried out by the solicitor in the process of negotiations to complete the sale have already been described on page 27. If you are selling your practice, the following advice may be useful:

a. Advertise the practice at a sensible price, then you will probably have a rush of viewers. Your first ones will most likely be the best.

b. You do not necessarily need an estate agent as you can sell the practice by placing an advertisement in one of the medical journals or periodicals.

c. Do make sure the practice is tidy and make a list of what you wish to sell and what constitutes fixtures and fittings. Use common sense to decide what may be useful to you in the future, for example, a car.

You are selling a most prized possession. You will have to work at selling it and expect some inconvenience. Do not be oversensitive to what the viewer says and remember to keep control of the amount of stress you are subjected to. Negotiate slowly and carefully with the help of the solicitor. He will deal with all the relevant documents, application forms, registry forms and contracts. The buyer will probably ask a lot of questions, but you can always ask him to rely on his own survey if you do not have an answer.

Making a will

This is a responsible action for your family and any other dependants who will have an interest in your private practice in the event of your death, not only in a single-handed practice but also in a partnership. There may be a clause in the agreement to buy the deceased partner out which will probably be of great assistance to your family. State all the facts carefully and make them as simple as possible.

Legacies

Occasionally, patients will show their appreciation of your services by leaving you a legacy in their wills. This can be a very vulnerable situation, and if you know that it might occur, it is advisable to insist that the patient seeks independent legal advice first. Any unpleasantness which may occur later is then avoided, and you are discharging your duty in the right way.

You may have to deal with the executors of a deceased patient or a deceased fellow partner, so make sure that at all times you act in a totally professional manner.

PRACTITIONER CHECK LIST

1. Are you aware of your ethical and legal responsibilities?
2. Do you know the professional rules of conduct?
3. Have you chosen the title of the practice?
4. Will you contact other practitioners to share a block booking in the Yellow Pages?
5. Have you composed the format of a letter to send to other practitioners announcing your availability?
6. Have you read the Data Protection Act 1984?
7. Have you taken out all the necessary insurances?
8. Do you really understand a partnership agreement?
9. Have you decided on how to share the profits?
10. Has the solicitor checked all the legal agreements with you?
11. Have you enough life assurance cover?
12. Have you made a will?

5

Office planning and management

All clean and comfortable, I sit down to write.
John Keats 1795–1821

THE OFFICE

Typing, filing and general secretarial and administrative duties form the main part of the work carried out in the office. In the past, little attention was paid to the requirements either of the office itself or the person doing the work.

Modern efficient medical practice demands that the importance of the office is recognised and that consideration is given both to its needs and those of the secretary or administrative assistant. Ideally, the office must be a separate room as it is the central focus for the practice administration and it forms a natural gathering place for the staff who need access to information, files, notice boards and records.

The secretary needs somewhere quiet to work without undue interruption in pleasant and well-planned surroundings. A good secretary is expensive and her worth must be reflected in the facilities which are provided.

The business office must be adequate in size. In a small practice, it may double as a rest room for the staff. Office space is always grossly underestimated or neglected in planning, which leads to overcrowding, poor working conditions and frayed tempers. As the practice develops more storage space will be required, and this must be allowed for when the practice is planned initially.

It has been estimated that approximately 11.25 m² (125 sq ft) of space is needed for each person using the room.

Office furniture

Office furniture will consist of:
1. A desk or table. This must be large enough to accommodate a

89

typewriter, telephones and maybe a computer, and still allow for sufficient working space.

2. A comfortable upright chair with adjustments for secretarial use.
3. Shelves.
4. A typewriter.
5. Telephone services.
6. Filing cabinets and files, both flat and of the box type.
7. Possibly a small computer.
8. A fire extinguisher.
9. Reference books.
10. A chair for staff or patients.

There must be good lighting, so the desk should be placed where natural daylight can be utilised, if possible. A well-balanced desk light is an asset. Shelving must be at a sensible height and the shelves must be wide enough to accommodate files, books and papers—18–20 cm (7–8 in) is a good width. Filing cabinets must be placed so there is enough space to open drawers. This all may seem obvious, but it is essential to have space. Keep the office arrangement flexible as you may well wish to change it in the future.

The staff room

The staff must have a room to change their clothes, if necessary, and separate washing and cloakroom facilities. They will need somewhere to relax and eat during off-duty periods in the day, so comfortable chairs and kitchen utensils must be provided. A kettle, toaster, small grill and a refrigerator are useful. The room must always be kept tidy and the door closed. Lockers or a cupboard with keys to leave handbags, briefcases or other valuables in safety are necessary.

Prevention of theft

Theft is an increasing problem. Patients' records can be stored in a fireproofed locked metal filing cabinet. A safe can be used for drugs which do not require refrigeration, money, important documents or patients' valuables which may be left behind by mistake after treatment. A small floor safe will probably be sufficient; it is a tax deductible expense and there are several firms offering such protection.

Fire extinguishers

A major fire is a disaster and can start so easily. However well you are insured, it is a worrying and distressing experience.

Fire precautions have already been mentioned in Chapter 2 and it will be necessary to have a fire certificate if you employ more than ten people anywhere other than on the ground floor (The Health and Safety At Work Act 1974 and the Fire Precautions Act 1971).

There are several classes of fire. Their classification depends on how they start—for example, from an electrical fault or from a carelessly discarded cigarette.

An investment in two or three of the following extinguishers from a reputable firm which can be recommended by the fire officer and the insurance broker, will be necessary:

1. An extinguisher which covers all classes of fire. This will contain a dry chemical mixture which does not cause considerable damage. Never use a water extinguisher on an electrical fire.
2. Fire buckets filled with either sand or water. All waste receptacles must be metal, as although they are not very attractive, they will contain a smouldering cigarette until it is noticed and something can be done about it.
3. A fire blanket to smother a small fire or wrap around a person.
4. Smoke detectors which are usually fitted on the ceiling and which emit a very loud noise when the smoke density reaches a certain level. As they are powered by batteries, they must be checked every three months.

Check also that the other extinguishers are still full, approximately every six months; they have a glass gauge for this purpose. The firm supplying the extinguishers will demonstrate to you and your staff how to use them and it is essential that every new member of staff is familiar with their use.

Storage areas

Allocating space for future storage is always neglected in office planning. Medical supplies, accessories, stationery, linen and books all have to be stored. When you start, it will not be seen as a major problem. Be warned, however: after years of accumulating paper, files and supplies, storage space suddenly becomes limited. Careful planning is, therefore, essential. Space is expensive so every nook and cranny must be utilised with cupboards, shelves or some type of storage unit.

BUYING OFFICE FURNITURE AND EQUIPMENT

It is worth checking with the local hospital and other practitioners in the area whether there is a firm offering special rates for providing furniture and office equipment. Sometimes the firm will offer a discount when you make your first large purchase.

Business office equipment

There are certain essential pieces of equipment which must be purchased.

1. *A typewriter*

Many practitioners have illegible handwriting! Typewritten letters and reports give a crisp, modern and professional image. If you can't afford an electric typewriter, then buy a good quality manual one. Typewriters are now available with word processors and computer memory banks. What you finally select will depend on your own individual practice, but electronic gadgetry is very expensive, so do not buy equipment you do not need and probably cannot use.

2. *A word processor*

This is a very useful piece of equipment. It can facilitate sending out accounts, writing letters, addressing envelopes, writing research papers and compiling reports.

3. *A calculator*

A calculator will make life much easier. Calculators range from very inexpensive models to those with complex functions which you probably do not need. It is advisable to buy one with a print out slip, as when you are working through a lot of calculations it is helpful to see what you have done. If you make a mistake, it is difficult to see where you have gone wrong if there is no record. Adding machines have print outs and are useful if there are a large number of financial figures to calculate, but it will not be necessary to have both an adding machine and a calculator.

4. *An office copier*

This piece of equipment is almost indispensable in some practices. It will copy patients' records, forms for insurance companies, letters, reports, patients' accounts and anything else which can be put on paper. Attention must be paid to the quality of reproduction when purchasing a copier, and the ability of the machine to cope rapidly with the originals.

Some models are designed for small businesses and fit on a shelf or desk top, but again they are fairly expensive and it may be necessary to wait until the practice needs one before investing the capital.

5. *Dictating machines*

Many practitioners find the flexibility of carrying portable dictating units extremely useful. They are small and lightweight and can be used inside or outside the practice and in the car. The tape from the machine can be easily passed on to a secretary for audio-typing, who can stop it, rewind and correct any errors, and the tape can then be re-used.

COMMUNICATIONS

Telephone services

A telephone is essential when you begin in private practice. No printing work can commence until the practice has an address and telephone number. If the practice has no existing telephone, apply for one as soon as you are certain the premises are yours. It will take several weeks to get a telephone installed, particularly in an area where the demand is heavy since there may be no free lines and you will have to wait until one becomes available. Generally, however, lines for business purposes are allocated fairly quickly.

It is certainly an advantage if you can afford two lines. If one is engaged, a worried patient or relative can use the other, and the telephone will not sound constantly engaged if you use one line only for outgoing calls. Two lines have another important advantage: if one is out of order the patients do have a second number to use. This is essential if there is an emergency.

Telephones can be bought or leased. The choice is personal and financial. If you are short of capital, it is wise to rent initially and buy when you know exactly what type of telephone system you want. Make sure a qualified engineer connects the telephone. It may be tempting to do it yourself, but if an amateur effort leads to an annoying buzz or a line which only works intermittently you will do neither yourself nor the practice any good at all.

A visit to the telephone company sales department to choose the equipment and obtain a listing in the local telephone directory is wise. It speeds up the process of filling in the appropriate forms and you can select the type and design of telephone, switchboard, intercom system, answering machine or any other device you require, on the spot.

Answering machines

When you first start in practice, you may be entirely on your own. You will need to find some way of taking calls even if you are out visiting patients. There is nothing more frustrating for the patient than an unanswered telephone.

An answering machine is, therefore, one of the solutions. It is less than ideal, since many people show a marked reluctance to use it, and its unpopularity may lead the patient to telephone another practitioner.

The message you leave on the machine must be brief, clear and of good quality. It should state where you are, when you will be back and request a message to be left for you. Encourage the caller to telephone you again—this saves making a long list of return calls when you get back.

If you leave the machine on over a weekend or holiday, make it quite clear that the practice is closed, but state when it will re-open. You can leave a referring number on the tape if you wish to take calls at home.

It is hoped that answering machines will become more acceptable as they are extremely useful. You can rent or buy the machine of your choice. Renting is the more practical option as the technology is improving all the time and if you have a fairly short rental agreement you can update your model regularly.

Answering service

If the volume of your incoming calls is likely to be heavy, and you do not wish to employ a receptionist, an answering service is an alternative method to an answering machine. The firm you use must be given some guidelines on how to monitor your particular calls, and how to categorise them in the best way possible. You should specify when you do not want to be called, your preference for accepting calls from other practitioners, and a number where help can be obtained if there is an emergency.

Call divertors

These machines are very useful if you are going to be away from the practice, but in one place for some time. They divert incoming calls to the practice to any number you programme into the machine. If you are on call at home, this is an obvious way to receive calls from the practice. They are, however, of limited use if you are constantly on the move, as it is not possible at the moment to re-programme the machine to divert calls to a different number, unless you go back to the practice to do it.

You will need two telephone lines to accommodate a divertor. The cost of the call once it has been diverted from the practice to wherever you are, is your responsibility.

Call systems

A patient sitting in the waiting room needs to be informed that the practitioner is ready to see him for consultation or treatment. This can be done in one of the following ways.
1. The practitioner or receptionist may come in person and call the next patient, but if it is a single-handed practice, this can be time-consuming and tiring.
2. A good intercom system can be installed from your room to either the waiting room or reception area where the receptionist can then call the next patient. This system has disadvantages as if you are single handed, patients who are hard of hearing do not always hear the calls. There is no doubt that a personal welcome is the best, but if you are extremely busy and wish to ensure the smooth running of the practice, you will have to use one of these systems.

Car telephones and cellular network

Car telephones have existed for some years and now have been revolutionised by the introduction of cellular communication. A subscriber is allocated an individual number, and this remains his number no matter where he or his car may be. As soon as he switches on the car telephone, his nearest switching centre monitors his call and assigns him an available frequency. There is no congestion in the channels, range is not limited and the strength and clarity is good. The country is divided into a network of areas or cells which vary in size, according to the expected numbers of subscribers within it. As a subscriber moves from area to area, he is automatically switched into the new cell. Cellular system prices are very competitive and are expected to come down as technology improves.

The top end of the cellular range models are designed so that they can be easily removed from the car and taken with the subscriber. These are still very expensive, and heavy, so it might be advisable to wait until they are cheaper and lighter.

In spite of all the contrivances to keep you in touch with the patient, there is something reassuring about a person at the other end of the telephone. If you cannot afford one of these methods, try and arrange your visiting out of normal practice hours. It can be very difficult to achieve, as a sick patient may need immediate attention and the visit may take longer than anticipated. The nagging anxiety about telephone calls when you are away from the practice must encourage you to choose and plan some method of having the telephone answered in your absence.

Yellow Pages and other directories

These are regional directories listing the specialities throughout the United Kingdom; certain other countries also have Yellow Pages. Each directory is reprinted annually. The rates for insertion vary with each directory according to the circulation, and a charge is made for each line other than the name, address, qualification and telephone number of the subscriber. Each directory has its own closing date for entries, so apply promptly. Establish whether there is a block booking with other practitioners which will make it easier for the patient when seeking treatment. (See Advertising, p. 76.)

FILING EQUIPMENT AND SYSTEMS

Filing equipment

There are two types of storage to choose from, unless you are using a computer:

1, *Open shelf filing*

This takes the form of open horizontal shelves for medical box files of various heights and widths. It is a relatively cheap form of filing and it can be assembled on available wall space in the office and increased as the practice grows.

2. *Closed cabinet and drawer filing*

These are constructed with a locking device, thus providing confidentiality and security against theft, dirt and dust. Make sure you put the spare key in a sensible place. There is nothing more embarrassing than losing the original and not being able to have access to the files. The drawers are of different heights and widths, and the files may be laterally or vertically placed inside. They are usually metal and come in various colours to blend with the decor, so it is not necessary to have battleship grey. They are obviously neater and tidier than open filing.

Filing systems and records

The method used will be determined by the requirements of the practice, cost and available space. Records take up a great deal of space.

The four most common categories are:
1. Alphabetical filing.
2. Numerical filing.
3. Colour coding.
4. Office charting.

Spelling and filing errors occur in alphabetical filing. It is also difficult to retrieve records of patients with commonly used surnames. It is wise to establish rules which should be followed by all the staff. The following key points may be useful:
1. The patient's surname, given name and initials must be filed in alphabetical order.
2. Lord, Sir, Mr, Mrs, and other titles should be disregarded.
3. Identification labels must be typed, not handwritten.
4. Identical surnames should be filed in order, by using the first or given name as the guide, i.e. Johnson Samuel is filed before Johnson Stephen.

In numerical filing each patient is given a sequential number. However, there has to be an alphabetical cross index if hundreds of records are stored.

Filing is tedious and time consuming, accuracy can be poor and any system needs to be updated and tidied up regularly. Careful thought and a good system will prevent files from being misfiled, mislaid or lost.

An alternative method is to store your records on a computer.

Computers

A computer system provides a method of storing information and producing it on demand. Information is usually put into the computer by means of a keyboard, but the introduction of touch screens, and particularly voice recognition systems, may well make the keyboard obsolete in the future. Information is produced either on a visual display unit or by means of a printout.

Essentially, all information which can be stored on paper, i.e., patients' records, financial data and personal details, can be stored by the computer. It is possible to programme the system to analyse data and produce it in a way which can provide indications of future patient numbers, the percentage of patients with any given condition and a forecast of the practice profits next year.

Before deciding to install a computer, it is important to consider the following points:

1. Do I really need a computer?
2. Is the volume of paperwork sufficient to justify the expense?
3. How many people will use it?
4. What systems are available with suitable programmes for the practice?
5. Who will need to be trained to use the computer?
6. Can I afford the initial outlay?
7. Can the capacity of the computer be upgraded without undue trouble in the future?
8. Are other practitioners using a similar system to the one I am considering and are they happy with it?
9. Will it alter the functions of the practice to everyone's benefit, or will it disrupt the routine to no good purpose?
10. Will it really contribute to the smooth running and efficient management of the practice?

The choice of computer

The eventual decision to purchase a computer and the choice of a suitable system will depend on the individual requirements of the practice. An unwary practitioner should not be tempted to buy an impressive system. It will be too sophisticated for the practice and will need highly specialised personnel to operate it; nor should too small a system be purchased as it is unlikely to have the storage facilities you require. When you have narrowed down your choice to two or three systems, ask the computer company to give you the names of at least one user in your area and check for yourself that it works well, performs the functions you require and is reliable.

Computer technology is changing very rapidly and it is important that the model you choose can be updated and that the accessories and programmes will be available for some time.

The supplier will offer a maintenance contract and normally provides service within 24 hours in case of a breakdown.

Computer hardware can be supplied as a compact desk top unit (Fig. 5.1) incorporating the following items:

1. Visual display unit—VDU.
2. A keyboard.
3. A disc storage unit.

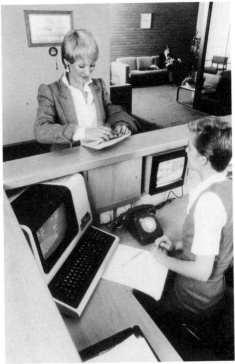

Fig. 5.1 A computer station.

4. The micro-processor.

The computer will store anything you wish, but it will mainly be used for:

1. The register of patients and their medical records.
2. The patients' treatment and results.
3. Information relating to the practice finances.
4. Statistical information.
5. Personal information.

The advantages of a computer

1. It performs logical operations at a high speed.
2. It will store a huge amount of data and records for the lifetime of patients, thus providing easy accessibility to this information.
3. Jobs can be tackled which would only be possible with a computer because of its versatility and flexibility.
4. It is accurate in relaying information in a partnership or group practice.

The disadvantages of a computer

1. A computer is expensive.
2. Errors may occur which can destroy a programme and this is costly.
3. The human errors can be disruptive.

Data protection

The object of the Data Protection Act 1984 is to protect the individual (data subject) from misuse of personal data held in a computer by the data user. Personal data as defined by the Act is: 'data consisting of information which relates to a living individual who can be identified from that information or from that and other information in possession of the data user'. Data is also defined as information recorded in a form in which it can be processed by equipment automatically in response to instructions given for that purpose. The equipment includes word processors, main frame, mini- and micro-computers. The Act further provides that any company, organisation or individual which is a user of personal information data falling within the definition of the Act and on equipment defined in the Act, must register with the Data Protection Registrar.

There are certain exemptions such as: 'any operation performed only for the purpose of preparing the text of documents'. Problems may arise in November 1987 when data subjects have the right of access to information held on them in a computer. At the present time there is no legislation to prevent a patient from having access to his clinical records as from 1987, although this situation could well change. It would be advisable for practitioners contemplating using a computer for this purpose to check with the Data Protection Registrar if and when a firm decision is made.

PRINTING AND STATIONERY

Once the title, name, address and telephone numbers of the practice have been established, you can start ordering your printed stationery. These requirements can be met either by a local printer or one who specialises in medical printing. Print shops also offer very good comprehensive services and because the method of printing is essentially photocopying, they may be quicker and possibly cheaper than a traditional printer. The printing must look professional, clear and uncluttered, and it must contain all the information you wish to convey.

Letterheads

You may decide to have a logo which becomes identified with the practice. Make sure it is well designed and appropriate. Printing must be on good quality paper which is usually white. The lettering may be of any colour, but black or blue are popular and look professional on white paper. The letterhead can be embossed or engraved with the logo, name, address and telephone number, but this is fairly expensive. You will need two sizes of paper: A4 which is suitable for long letters and records and A5 for shorter letters. A second unheaded sheet of paper for longer letters and reports with matching envelopes for both sizes of paper, will also be required.

Professional cards

These are essential and are usually printed on thin lightweight card. Different type styles can be chosen and they can be printed or engraved. Many practitioners use the same form as their letterheads to include the name, qualifications, address, telephone number and the hours the practice is open (see Fig. 5.2).

James D. West MCSP
Chartered Physiotherapist

2 Station Road   Hours 9.00 a.m. – 6.00 p.m.
Turville
Telephone No. 026 467321

Fig. 5.2 A professional card.

Appointment cards

These are similar in design and size to the professional cards. They must have spaces for writing in the patient's next appointment and follow-up times. It is worth stating the practice regulations on the card if a patient does not attend and has not telephoned to cancel the appointment within 24 hours (see Fig. 5.3).

Account forms

These will probably have the same letterhead as the notepaper, but

WESTCLIFFE CLINIC

3 Somerset Road
Westcliffe GH1 2BW
Westcliffe 312448

Will be pleased to see ....

on .... the .... at ....

on .... the .... at ....

on .... the .... at ....

PLEASE GIVE 24 HOURS NOTICE IF APPOINTMENT IS NOT REQUIRED, OTHERWISE A FEE WILL BE CHARGED

Fig. 5.3 An appointment card.

set out with sufficient space so that information such as what the account is for, the dates of attendance and the fee which is being charged, can be included.

Medical record cards

The method of recording consultations and treatment will vary according to the speciality and preference of the practitioner. It is advisable to use hard-wearing extra thick paper or thin card which can be stapled or filed in folders if necessary. The following general guidelines for the type and format of records may be useful:
1. The notes must be clear, concise and up-to-date, so simple, easy-to-read printing is necessary for any headings.
2. Some practices allow patients to fill in their names, age and address to save time.
3. Questions if they are printed, must be simple and concise. For example: 'Do you frequently have nausea, vomiting or back pain', may be better asked:

Do you have back pain?	Yes .... No..........
How often?	....
Do you suffer from nausea?	Yes .... No..........
How often?	....

An appointment book

There are many ways of running an appointment system, but a book is the most commonly used method. It is possible to have one specially designed and printed, but this is very expensive. An appointment book which can be purchased from a good stationer will probably meet your requirements. Buy one which is large enough. The book must have plenty of space for each day for the patients' appointments, alterations which will inevitably occur, and any short notes you may wish to make. A pencil and rubber must accompany the book.

Name and address book

Keep a record of the names, addresses and telephone numbers of practitioners, suppliers, trades people, insurance companies, banks, professional advisers and hospitals, in a hard-backed indexed book. It is extremely helpful to make a note of everyone you deal with as you never know when you will need them again. This book must be kept near the telephone.

Memo pads

These are essential for recording telephone calls, jotting down quick reminders or leaving messages for the staff. Try and avoid putting down important bits of information on pieces of paper or the backs of envelopes—you will certainly mislay something important.

Rubber stamps and labels

You will find it convenient to use rubber stamps for various purposes. They are inexpensive and can usually be purchased from the local stationer. They can be custom-made, and as your practice develops you may find more uses for them. Some of the types of stamps you should have are as follows:
1. 'Received with thanks', for receipting paid accounts.
2. A date stamp with the name and address of the practice.
3. One with the logo of the practice.

Labels are also useful and the soft adhesive ones can be purchased from your locaL stationer and used for noting the service dates on pieces of medical equipment and supplies, fragile goods and marking important documents.

Office sundries

A noticeboard, a stapler, pens, biros, drawing pins, paper clips, sellotape, pencils and a pencil sharpener, a paper knife and a pair of scissors will all be required.

The mail and postage

It is important to have somewhere to put the mail. Trays in various colours are a good idea. You can then have one for accounts paid, one for bills to be paid, another for advertising material, and an IN and OUT tray for medical correspondence and reports. This will avoid confusion. You will have to handle and reply to some of the correspondence on a daily basis, so do not forget to allow time. Keep a plentiful supply of stamps of all values in the office drawer.

REFERENCE BOOKS

The following list of books for the office and staff room are only a few suggestions which may be helpful. You will wish to update them or buy more when the practice expands:

1. A standard English dictionary. Poor or incorrect spelling gives a very bad impression. If you are not certain about the spelling of a word, look it up.
2. A standard medical dictionary. This will be especially useful for any non-medical members of staff who type letters or reports.
3. Relevant professional directories.
4. Your own medical textbooks.
5. Telephone directories, code books and Yellow Pages directories.
6. Postage rates and directories.
7. Local trade directories.
8. A first aid handbook.
9. An office handbook.
10. This book, of course!

TRANSPORTATION AND THE CAR

The purchase of a car will most probably be necessary in running the business, particularly if you are visiting domiciliary patients. Motoring is expensive and the subsequent running costs are an important and heavy overhead. A reliable car is indispensable. Every practice has its share of patients who need to be seen in their homes. In a rural practice you may have to spend time and energy travelling long distances in all weathers. It can prove expensive, therefore, in terms of your time as well as in petrol or fares. A car must be chosen that is economic in its consumption of petrol and capable of taking equipment and supplies, if necessary. Hatchbacks are very popular, as it is easier to move equipment in and out of a spacious hatchback car than a small boot. The car must be serviced regularly by a local reputable garage. Try and have a permanent space allocated for parking outside the practice in the city and the country, so that you can get to it quickly in an emergency. In some cities, it is advisable to hire a taxi to avoid parking delays, strain and frustration.

The cost of running a car is formidable and not always

appreciated at the time it is purchased. It may have to be used for both the family and the practice, or it may be a matter of agreement between partners as to how a car for the practice is purchased.

In some practices, the purchase is the responsibility of each partner; in others the partnership owns the cars and makes finance available for their purchase.

The second method may be preferable as it usually ensures that all the partners have reliable cars that are regularly serviced. The total value of the cars will appear in the partners' capital accounts (see Ch. 3). If a partner leaves, sometimes a car is used in part payment of the share of the capital, therefore relieving the liquidity of the practice.

Buying the car

Before you buy a car, consider the following points:
1. Do I really need one for the practice? If you are in a city, using a taxi or hiring a car may prove cheaper than running one. If it sits in the garage, it is costing you money.
2. Spend time deciding what type of car you want.
3. Make sure you have the available finance to buy and insure the car. It is essential it is as burglar-proof as possible.
4. If you use a dealer, check that he is reputable and reliable. Join one of the motoring organisations who may prove very useful in the event of a breakdown.

Running costs of the car

Once you drive the car away from the showroom or garage the following costs will occur:
1. Petrol costs.
2. Road fund licence.
3. Insurance.
4. Depreciation.
5. Repairs, replacements and servicing.
6. Motoring organisation subscriptions.
7. Car parking fees, meters and the inadvertent fines.

Make sure you get maximum use from the car for the minimum amount of capital outlay.

PRACTITIONER CHECK LIST

1. Do the staff have adequate space and facilities?
2. Are the fire extinguishers full and in position?
3. Is storage space being used to full capacity?
4. Have you efficient security?
5. Have you chosen a method of filing and storage for the office?
6. Have you two telephone lines for a more efficient reception system.
7. Can future information storage requirements be accommodated in a computer?
8. Are the displays and printouts clear?
9. Will a logo be suitable for letterheads for the practice?
10. Is the paper you have chosen for medical records suitable for a period of years?
11. Is it time to have a telephone in the car?

6

Practice planning and management

Be not the first by whom the new are tried
Nor yet the last to lay the old aside.
Alexander Pope 1688–1744

Some time must be spent planning the layout and appearance of the practice. It must be practical, professional and comfortable. A balance must be struck between too clinical an image which can be unwelcoming and a decorative scheme which is unsuitable for professional practice.

In general, the decor should reflect the practice surroundings. If it is in an elegant and dignified house you will need to consider a more traditional approach to decoration than if the practice is in a very modern building with large wide picture windows and the extensive use of exposed brickwork.

DECOR

The practice decor must project a professional image. Interior designers and decorators are expensive, but if you do not have a good, imaginative sense of colour and design, then you will need the help of a spouse, a friend or a professional.

The colour scheme

Colour schemes can create the illusion of space. Light colours will make a room seem larger, and rich warm tones, such as orange, brown and coral, give a feeling of warmth. Pale blues and greens are tranquil and restful, but they can be cold. Patterned wallpaper can be used for the reception area, providing it is attractive and simple. It is more practical to paint treatment areas. Pictures can be a useful asset in addition to the colour scheme, especially in the reception room where patients are waiting. They often provide an interest and a talking point with other patients.

Furnishings

The furnishings in the reception area and office should be attractive, comfortable and functional. They should be well made and the colours should co-ordinate with the rest of the decor. Chairs should be of varied heights to suit the patients' requirements. The material and surface tops to tables should be well polished or of a material that is easily maintained. Tables should not be too low.

Floor coverings

The floor covering should be attractive and easy to clean, and require minimum maintenance. It should be non-slip and warm on the feet. A commercial grade of wall-to-wall carpeting can be attractive. This can be the best choice for the reception area, hallways and consultation rooms, providing there will not be frequent spillages on the floor. Carpeting is expensive, but it is worth buying a good quality carpet to start with as certain areas of the practice will take a lot of wear. In some professions, linoleum, cork, rubber, plastic or terrazo tiles may provide a better and more practical choice of covering for the floor.

Walls and partitions

Walls and partitions should be sound-proofed if you are going to respect the privacy of the patient. A curtained-off area is not really satisfactory if the patient wishes to speak to you in confidence. Many practitioners and private hospitals only use curtains for dividing treatment areas. This does not allow complete privacy and is not recommended if a high standard of patient care and confidentiality is to be provided.

Partitions can be rather flimsy, but they can be easily erected and glass partitioning at the top will allow more light into the room.

Corridors, passages and stairs

These must be wide enough to allow two people to pass each other comfortably. 1.5 m (5 ft) is an ideal width and will give room for a wheelchair to pass. They should also have a non-slip surface, and the stairs should have a good strong handrail. Handicapped patients and those on crutches will thank you for care over these points.

Windows, curtains and blinds

Windows must be clean in order to give a hygienic clinical image. Blinds are less of a dust trap than curtains, and vertical ones are more easily cleaned. Curtain material with a pattern to blend with the decor may be more cheerful and welcoming in the reception room windows and the office, and also around changing cubicles in the treatment rooms. A good window cleaner on a regular basis, which will mean one cheque or a petty cash payment, is desirable.

Lighting and mirrors

There must be adequate lighting, and enough mirrors in the reception room, consulting and treatment rooms, and cloakroom. Apart from giving an overall effect of space, mirrors are necessary for the patients' personal use and may be useful clinically in certain professions. A good table lamp can supplement the overhead lighting. Lamps should not be too large, but attractive and give a warm discreet light. Dimmer switches can be used to control the lighting in the treatment rooms if the patient is going to be discomforted by a continuous glare in his eyes.

Heating and ventilation

A feeling of warmth must pervade the practice. It is not pleasant to come into a practice or surgery on a cold wet foggy day only to find that there is inadequate heating and the practice is damp, draughty and chilly. Central heating should be installed if possible, and this can be boosted by an electric fire or fan heater when necessary. If there is a fireplace in the reception room and it is not used, an artificial fire will provide a warm welcoming glow.

In hot conditions, good air conditioning is essential. You must make sure that the atmosphere is not stuffy and the ventilation is adequate. However, open windows reduce privacy, increase noise from a busy road and allow in a great deal of dust and dirt.

The front door

The patient gets his first impression from the front door and nameplate when he arrives at the practice. A dignified and professional front door with a large letter box for all the mail, such as periodicals, sales literature, newspapers and magazines, is essential. A pleasant serviceable bell that works properly is important. If the building is occupied by practitioners other than yourself, the bell must be clearly marked so the patient does not have to guess which one is yours.

The front door must be wide enough for wheelchairs, stretchers and disabled patients. If there are steps, a ramp must be provided.

Nameplates

Nameplates are made from copper, brass, or other alloys, or from some form of plastic composition. They must be professional, discreet and always clean. The plate can be professionally engraved on a good quality base. Many department stores now offer engraving services, but the result is not always consistent and the plate itself can be thin. A professional engraver will use a good quality plate and the lettering will be of a high standard. Although this method may be more expensive, it is better to have the nameplate done properly at the beginning, and it will probably prove more weather-resistant. The plate must specify the name, letters of qualification and the profession which is practised, in accordance with the profession's rules of conduct.

A cleaner

A dirty, dusty and untidy practice is not pleasant. It presents a very poor image and gives an impression of carelessness. Cleaning must be done daily by a reliable person. All surfaces must be spotlessly clean and polished, the floor hoovered, plants watered, magazines and papers tidied, linen changed and waste baskets emptied.

However early you start in the morning, make sure all the cleaning is completed by the time the first patient arrives. A good daily can be hard to find, so you may have to consider using a commercial cleaning firm. Find out how much they charge for the work you want done and check the quality and reliability of their work with somebody else who is using their service. If you fail to find anybody to do the cleaning, you will have to do it yourself!

THE RECEPTION ROOM/WAITING AREA

Depending on your type of practice, this area may occupy a large proportion of the premises. If space is limited, the waiting area and reception desk can be in the hall. The seating and the size of the area must be adequate, not only for the patients, but also for the relatives and friends they frequently bring with them. It is an odd fact that strangers do not like sitting next to each other, so a larger area than you perhaps first envisaged is required (see Fig. 6.1). Planners usually recommend that if you see four patients in an hour, you

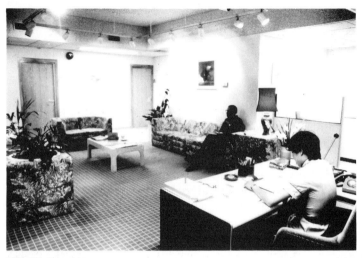

Fig. 6.1 Reception area.

should have twelve seating spaces in an area of approximately 16.2 m² (180 sq ft), in other words, three times the seating capacity for the number of individuals you have scheduled to see in the hour. Obviously, this is not always possible, but avoid couches and provide well-made sturdy attractive single seating units with good spinal support; often, banquette seating is used if space is limited. If you have room, a couch for a non-ambulant patient is desirable. However, he may be more comfortable on a mobile stretcher, in his wheelchair or in a spare treatment room. Do not leave him waiting in a draughty passage.

Coats, hats and umbrellas

There should be a space in the waiting room which is set aside for patients to leave their coats, hats and umbrellas. A stand for umbrellas is necessary.

Magazines

A rack or table carrying an adequate supply of general interest magazines is essential. There are companies which provide a regular subscription service for businesses. This is convenient as you make one order, write one cheque and have one renewal date. Obviously, you should also provide a cross-section of daily national newspapers.

Do not let your magazines become dusty, torn and two or three years out of date. You will not be enhancing the image of the practice.

Flowers

Flowers and plants in tasteful arrangements have a welcoming effect. Silk flowers and plants are a good way of avoiding continual worry about watering, providing they are not allowed to become drab and dusty. There are plenty of firms in the major towns and cities who offer a regular flower and plant service for businesses. This again means one order and one cheque on a regular basis.

Music

Background music is popular with some practitioners. It can provide a pleasant and relaxing atmosphere for patients who are sometimes tense when they arrive. However, continuous music, unless it is discreet and well chosen, can become an unpleasant, unwelcome and noisy throb.

Drinks

Have a supply of tea, coffee and soft drinks for your patients and visitors. A supply of drinking water should always be available.

Play items for children

A collection of small toys and children's books is a good idea to prevent boredom or upset at unfamiliar surroundings.

THE RECEPTIONIST/SECRETARY

This may be you or a member of your family at first. It is a key role in a practice and one from which the patients gain their first impressions. A friendly, sympathetic, relaxed, and calm person is ideal and one of the most important assets of the practice.

A good telephone manner and secretarial skills are essential. Many receptionists are very protective, but they must be trained properly, their duties clearly defined and they must always put the patient's interests first. If the practitioner is delayed, a courteous, helpful receptionist will put the patient at ease. A patient must never feel or be neglected, nor must he be kept waiting longer than necessary without a polite explanation.

Telephone reception

The telephone is usually the first point of contact with the practice for the patient and it is vital that calls and messages are dealt with carefully and efficiently.

The following guidelines may be of help:

1. Some practices have a standard printed form on which to put the name, address, telephone number and a brief outline of the patient's problem. These are quite helpful as it is possible to see at a glance the substance of the call.
2. Many patients wish to know your fees, the duration of treatment, methods of payment, whether a domiciliary service is offered, etc. Keep the call as short as you can without being discourteous: take the relevant details and a number you can use if you find it necessary to contact the patient.
3. Screening calls is a problem. You should not speak to a member of the family, another practitioner or patient when you are in the middle of a consultation. The patient is paying for your time and attention, and will not like interruptions.
4. An emergency call must be dealt with as soon as possible. Establish what the problem is, and decide what you are going to do about it.
5. Train the receptionist or secretary to distinguish between urgent and non-urgent calls.
6. If another practitioner telephones, it is polite to receive the call at the time whenever possible, but it will mean leaving your patient and disrupting the consultation.
7. A telephone line should be available for the patient's use as they will often wish to ring their office or home. Try and establish that they are not making long distance business calls by courtesy of your telephone bill. The telephone is best situated in the reception area, then no one patient can monopolise it.
8. Leave your own calls, either personal or business, to a time set aside for the purpose. Telephone reception can make or mar the reputation of the practice. As you get busier it will not be possible for you to see patients and answer the telephone, so it will be necessary to employ somebody.

Information notices

Attractive information signs are extremely useful since they help direct the patient and save a lot of questions. Many signs are mass produced by firms, or you can have them custom designed.

Such examples include:

1. No smoking. Please be considerate of other patients.
2. Fees are payable on completion of treatment.
3. Appointments not cancelled within 24 hours will be chargeable.
4. Important. If you wear a pacemaker, please inform the practice before treatment.
5. Car parking:
   a. Please park in the spaces provided.
   b. Please do not obstruct other vehicles.

CONSULTING OR TREATMENT ROOMS

Some consulting and treatment rooms are used by more than one practitioner. The room often becomes stamped with the personality of the practitioner. This is where the work is done and the room must give an overall welcoming effect. A pleasant setting with the clinical components required by the practitioner will require a minimum space of 8.64 m² (96 sq ft). A time and motion study has shown that three treatment rooms are the ideal number for a medium-sized practice.

The following are essential pieces of furniture for a consulting room:

1. An examination or treatment couch, preferably hydraulic.
2. A washbasin.
3. A waste receptacle.
4. A chair for both the patient and the practitioner.
5. A writing surface.
6. Storage cupboards.

The patient must have a small private area in which to change. A simple curtained-off space in one corner is adequate; or screens may be used if curtaining is not possible.

The medical equipment used professionally will dictate the amount of floor space you require. For example, dental practitioners and physiotherapists use large pieces of equipment, so each room must be tailored to meet the individual practitioner's requirements. Make sure you have sufficient power points for electrical equipment. Flex trailing across the floor is a hazard for everyone. The power points can be at waist level to avoid continual bending.

Linen and professional attire

A plentiful supply of good quality linen such as towels, sheets, pillow cases and blankets, either in white or colours which tone with the decor, are needed. Regular and frequent changing is necessary to maintain the highest possible standards of hygiene. Find a good local laundry, check their rates and pay the account monthly. Alternatively, a reliable washing machine and dryer can reduce laundry costs. Some practitioners use strong paper towelling instead of linen and this is now quite acceptable.

If white coats or tunics are worn these must be crisp, clean and changed daily.

Consultations

1. *Patients*

Patients are concerned about their symptoms. They do not know what to expect when they come to see you. They probably have ideas and are asking questions such as:
1. What is wrong with me?
2. What is the prognosis?
3. What is the practitioner going to do about it?

Use simple questions in your consultations. If the patient is evasive or unforthcoming, try and give him a lead so that you can control the way the information is given. This will establish his confidence and he will trust you. Listen to what the patient says: it will tell you a lot about him. Try and avoid using too much medical jargon: it will confuse and frighten the patient. Explain with drawings if it will help.

Do not leave a consultation or treatment with questions still unanswered. The patient must be aware of what is wrong with him, so that he can co-operate in appropriate actions and participate in decision-making. Proper management will benefit both the patient and the practitioner, and the responsibilities will be shared.

Make sure the patient is committed to what you advise; if he is not, find out why. However good your relationship with a patient may be, do not feel insulted if he does not return.

Your private practice will succeed if you constantly feed back

How regularly do you assess your clinical judgement and take a mental inventory of your work with patients. As an active clinician in private practice it should be routine.

Look at the following points carefully:

1. Analyse each patient's condition to identify specific problems with which your services will be concerned.

2. Establish specific goals which you hope to achieve in relation to each problem.

3. Specify measurable targets for the minimum level of success in achieving each goal you consider necessary for your services to be judged effective.

4. Consider more than one approach to the management of each problem.

5. Select the approach you use by following therapeutic guidelines which predict which method(s) will probably be safest and most effective based on key factors in the patient's history and present condition.

6. Make periodic measurements which give you objective evidence of the patient's progress towards each therapeutic and/or preventative goal.

7. Review the patient's rate of progress at regular intervals to decide whether your present programme of services is achieving satisfactory results, or needs to be revised.

8. Record your measurements of individual patients' problems and progress in such a way that data for many patients can be pooled and/or compared.

9. Consider the results you usually achieve with each type of patient you see frequently to decide whether your services are worthwhile.

10. Propose practical ways in which you believe your services could be made generally more effective by altering the methods you use or the timing and/or the location of your services.

Fig. 6.2 Self-assessment chart (reproduced by kind permission of Professor Nancy Watts, Massachusetts General Hospital, USA)

ideas tactfully, sympathetically and helpfully. Nothing must be taken for granted. The self-assessment chart (see Fig. 6.2) may help you assess your clinical work with your patients.

2. Treating other professionals

Professional custom will dictate your policy regarding the treatment of other practitioners. You will have to decide how to manage these circumstances. You can either extend professional courtesy and make no charge at all, or you may choose to treat at a very nominal amount. Many practitioners are covered for medical treatment by one of the insurance schemes. In this case, prepare an account in the normal way: the patient will not then feel awkward or guilty about not paying or having to reciprocate in some fashion. It is true that most practitioners do not expect treatment for nothing, but it is an area where there are few guidelines and the decision is left to the individual.

3. Discharging or terminating a patient's treatment

It is good practice to treat a patient, restore him to health and then discharge him. However, there are patients who just do not fit into this convenient timetabling. Discharging a patient who is not better and is unlikely to improve substantially is very difficult, particularly if he is relying on you psychologically rather than clinically. A gentle suggestion that a 'rest period' from treatment may be helpful as it prevents the patient from feeling he is 'cut off' and totally discharged; it also gives him an opportunity to resume treatment at a later stage if he wishes. The clinical decision to continue treatment is one which must be made by the individual practitioner based on the circumstances of the case. It may be wise to refer the patient to another type of practice or suggest an alternative form of treatment. These patients can present a dilemma, and care must be taken not to harass or upset the patient.

It is as well to send the patient an account for the treatment given. If it is appropriate, make it clear that it is an 'interim' account: this will help the patient feel he is still linked to the practice which may be very important for him.

With luck these difficulties will not occur, but forewarned is forearmed.

BUYING MEDICAL EQUIPMENT

The financial aspects of buying and leasing medical equipment have been discussed in a previous chapter. However, outright purchase is the best option if the capital is available.

Most manufacturers will let you have the equipment on trial for a month or two. This is extremely useful if you are contemplating buying one of the more expensive pieces of equipment. It need not necessarily be new, but you must take care to ensure that any second-hand items are sound. This means that the equipment must be in good mechanical order, and if it is a piece of electrical equipment, it must be completely safe.

In order to identify your needs, consider the anticipated caseload and your referral sources. Evaluate the equipment you need. If you are unsure, ask other practitioners. Try not to buy anything superfluous. Cost out the equipment you need and develop a list of priorities. The most essential items must head the list followed by the equipment you will want to add as your income becomes more supportive of the practice.

If you specialise, you may wish to purchase further equipment, but remember that it all has to be paid for.

Manufacturing and pharmaceutical companies

It is a good idea to compare prices from local sources as well as national companies, in order to establish which firms are the most competitive. You will be swamped initially with brochures of equipment, followed by frequent calls from representatives and medical suppliers, hoping to sell their company's products. These representatives provide an important and valuable service since they will keep you informed of what is new on the market and give you some research statistics which will back up their product's claims and draw attention to its side-effects and contra-indications. The good companies provide medical equipment very quickly in an emergency, and they will often lend a replacement whilst equipment is being repaired.

A note of warning: see the sales representatives by appointment only. The casual salesman who drops into the practice in the hope of persuading you to buy a piece of equipment in a weak moment must be discouraged. Besides wasting valuable time and disturbing your routine, it also gives the practice the wrong image.

Be courteous and offer a cup of coffee or tea, but state that an appointment is necessary so that he does not also waste his time sitting around waiting to see you.

Where to buy equipment

Regular articles on modern equipment are featured in the most popular medical journals, and equipment can be purchased directly from the manufacturer or from a major department store. Most medical conferences and meetings now run an exhibition of medical equipment. Visiting these exhibitions is a good way of seeing products if you are contemplating spending more capital on new equipment, and will prove worthwhile in terms of saving time and energy.

The service engineer

In certain professions, where a large amount of electrical apparatus is used, the service engineer plays an important role. He must be contacted immediately if something is at fault. Many companies offer a 24-hour service.

A friendly engineer who comes promptly can save your practice time and money. Electrical equipment must be serviced once a year and a certificate verifying that all of it is in order may be necessary for licensing and insurance purposes.

SCHEDULING PATIENTS' APPOINTMENTS

Initially, you may only see a few patients each day. They should be given appointments close together, so that one patient leaves as another arrives. You will then get into the habit of planning efficiently right from the beginning, and to the patient it will appear that you have a busy, thriving practice.

The time taken to see a patient will vary from practice to practice, depending on your profession and whether it is a first assessment, a consultation or follow-up treatment. Some practitioners will see six to eight patients in an hour; others will only schedule one or two new ones in an hour, with follow-up appointments for others. This gives both practitioner and patients time to be at ease with one another and does not make the patient feel he is being hurried.

The appointment system you choose will affect your entire practice management. Appointment books or diaries can be bought with timed appointments already set out, or it is possible to have your own books printed. The following guidelines may help you run your practice more smoothly and efficiently:

1. Be on time. If you are always late, the patient will go elsewhere.
2. Allow additional time for elderly or disabled patients, who may take a long time to get dressed or undressed, and for those who are very talkative.
3. Patients attending for the first time will take longer as their history must be recorded, an assessment made and treatment may be necessary.
4. Emergency patients will throw out your scheduling, but they must be seen.
5. If you know a patient is habitually late, give him an appointment half-an-hour before the scheduled time. This usually works, but he may surprise you!
6. Do not be put out by the patient who arrives very early: see him at the correct appointed time. If you see him before he will always expect it.
7. Check the appointment book regularly to make sure a helpful member of staff or enthusiastic receptionist has not overbooked your time.
8. If a patient walks in off the street and wants to be seen at once,

---

Mr D. Pearce   **The Dental Clinic**
BDS LDS RCS   01 731 5341

                                          September 1985

Mrs P. Thompson,

This is to remind you that it is now 6 months since your last dental

treatment.

At your request, I am reminding you that should you wish to make

an appointment, please contact my receptionist at the above

telephone number.

Fig. 6.3 Patient reminder card (see p. 122).

give him an appointment even if he has to return later in the day.

9. Indicate on your appointment card that you reserve the right to charge for cancelled appointments if the practice is not notified 24 hours in advance.

10. Send reminder notices if they are appropriate.

Patient reminders

It is unethical to solicit a patient's return to the practice, but certain professions remind patients of follow-up appointments.

The following suggestions may be helpful:

1. *Telephone calls*

24–48 hours before the scheduled time of the patient's appointment, you or a member of staff should telephone the patient to remind him of the appointment. Ask for a telephone number at work so the calls can be made during the day and not in the evening.

2. *Appointment cards*

A printed appointment card setting out the details of the appointment date and time may be given to the patient.

3. *Mailing reminders*

Some practices ask patients to fill in their name and address on a card which can be posted to them at the appropriate time (see Fig. 6.3). This is quite acceptable and falls within the bounds of medical etiquette.

ACCOUNTS: METHOD AND COLLECTION

Fees

Patients must always be aware, at the outset, of the fee for a proposed consultation or treatment and the likely number of appointments which may be necessary. If you envisage a long period of treatment, you must warn the patient, particularly if he is going to pay his own account. In certain cases, an interim account must be rendered to prevent the amount reaching too high a level.

Rendering the account

Your service is free until it is paid for. Some suggestions for successful collections are:

1. Inform the patient at the first visit how the accounts are settled. This may be at each attendance by cash, cheque or a credit card.
2. If you do not have a secretary or a receptionist, and find it difficult to discuss money with the patient, give him a leaflet on the first visit which explains and states the method of paying and the scale of the fees.
3. If the patient is covered by a medical insurance scheme, an account will be given at the end of a course of treatment. Ask the patient for his medical scheme policy number to ensure its validity. Many patients now use a credit card system for claiming their medical insurance accounts.
4. The account must be clearly itemised, with the dates of treatment and any extras, such as medical supplies or equipment.
5. Accounts must be sent regularly, either weekly or at the end of each month. If an account remains unpaid, and you have to re-issue a bill, a handling charge can be made.
6. Use a coloured envelope for sending out accounts. Studies indicate this is more likely to elicit payment than accounts sent in a brown envelope!
7. Use regular reminder notices for persistent slow payers.

   Fortunately, the majority of patients pay their accounts promptly but there are always a few who refuse to settle their bills, despite polite reminders. A patient who does not pay provides the practice with a loss. When you have exhausted all the usual methods to obtain settlement, there are several remaining options open to recover the debts.

Credit cards

Credit cards have become an important development in borrowing money to pay accounts. They are issued by the clearing banks. If they are used properly, they can be extremely useful when you plan your spending since you can choose the method and timing of the repayments. They are also used by certain medical insurance companies and patients for paying your professional fees.

1. *A personal or practice credit card*

The interest rate on the credit will vary with the bank rate. The bank will decide how much credit it will give you and this is usually a fixed amount. The credit card has the advantage of eliminating the need for cash or a cheque when you are buying different items. Make sure you do not mix up personal purchases with any practice items when you use your credit card as it will only lead to confusion in the accounting records.

2. *Credit cards in payment of fees*

The advantages of payment by credit card are:
a. It is convenient for the patients.
b. Since immediate payment is received, it improves the cash flow of the practice.
c. It reduces the collection of overdue accounts or bad debts, since these are transferred to the credit card company.

The disadvantages of the credit card system include the following:
 (i) Use of credit cards is not always considered professional.
 (ii) The service charge levied by the bank or credit card company reduces the fee you collect from the patient.
(iii) The bank or credit card company will still charge a service amount even if no payments take place by credit card during any one month.

The banks and credit card companies issue the charge tickets, imprinting machines and all the necessary documentation and identification materials. Make sure that if you pay for any practice items by credit card, payment is recorded in the usual way in the practice books. If payment is by personal credit card, do ensure that the practice pays you back.

Credit control

Debt collection

Bad debts may be recovered by one of the following methods:

1. *A solicitor's letter.* This form of account collecting is best used in the first instance, but it can be expensive. It has the advantage that a letter from a solicitor usually produces quick results.

2. *A commercial debt collecting agency.* There are many agencies

which specialise in the collection of medical fees. It is important to choose one with a good reputation. Check the promptness with which the agency settles payment and the percentage they charge for each account collected. Normally a detailed statement and cheque is sent to the client each month.

3. *The small claims division of the local county court.* These courts have been established to handle claims involving small sums of money. The advantages of this system are that it is not necessary to use the services of a lawyer, and the procedure is relatively simple. A form setting out the details of the claim is filled in, and the appropriate fee for filing the claim is paid—this is normally a percentage of the total amount outstanding which is recoverable from the debtor. These and copies of the outstanding bills are left with the court. The practitioner does not have to appear in court. The court officers send a copy of the claim to the debtor, who will normally settle the account at this stage. If he does not, then the court will take further action to obtain satisfaction. If the account is disputed, the case is referred to the court for a decision which is binding on both parties. This method of collecting accounts has the advantage that the order to pay issued by the court will seldom if ever be ignored. Its disadvantage is that the practitioner has to initiate the early stages himself which can be time consuming. A booklet explaining the procedure for the recovery of debts can be obtained from the local county court.

4. *Large debts above a certain amount which are not within the jurisdiction of the county court, will be recovered by an action in the High Court.* This is an undesirable situation as you will need the services and help of a lawyer to take an action to the High Court. It is a complicated and slow procedure. Try, therefore, to avoid overdue or outstanding accounts becoming too high.

There must be a professional approach in debt recovery and credit control. Bad debts can seriously affect the profits of the practice and it is vital to maintain a good cash flow and adequate working capital. Follow up patients promptly and firmly, by reminders and telephone calls if necessary. No harassment or abusive techniques must be used in collecting outstanding accounts or tracing the absconding debtor.

Tracing a patient

A patient may change his address without paying the bill. A number of things can be done to settle the account:

1. Request the new correct forwarding address from the Post Office who will usually have it, but you may have to pay a small charge to have the accounts re-directed.
2. Telephone the patient's family and inquire about the patient's new address.
3. Contact the family general practitioner for forwarding details as he will have had to send the medical records to a new location.
4. Contact the patient's place of work. Do not state the purpose of the inquiry. The firm may be reluctant to disclose any details since it is the policy of many firms not to give any information.

Death

If a patient dies owing you money, you may not wish to pursue the matter further. If you do, however, wish to recover your account, the following steps can be taken:

1. Send a copy of the account to the patient's next of kin. It can then either be paid or passed on to the executor of the deceased's estate. The required formalities will have to be observed by the executor, so it may take some time for the settlement to be forthcoming.
2. If the patient is covered by medical insurance, send the account at once to the company.
3. Contact the patient's bank who may be handling the outstanding claims at the time of the patient's death. The address of the bank will be given to you by the deceased's executor.

If the practitioner should die and a spouse has to collect the outstanding fees, this should be handled along with other matters relating to the practice, by an accountant and a solicitor. There will be a number of legal and tax implications which must be dealt with by professional advisers.

PRACTITIONER CHECK LIST

1. Is the floor surface safe for the patients?
2. Do the patients have complete privacy to talk in confidence?
3. Is the practice warm enough?
4. Is there adequate ventilation?
5. Are the doorways and corridors wide enough?
6. Have you arranged for information notices to be made?
7. Is your telephone reception satisfactory?

8. Have you found a reliable service engineer?
9. Is the linen clean?
10. Have you a patient reminder system?
11. Is your credit control producing results?
12. Is the practice so busy that you now need extra staff and space?

7

Personnel and hospital management

Patiently adjust, amend and heal.
Thomas Hardy 1840–1928

EMPLOYING STAFF

The most obvious reason for employing staff and sharing responsibility is to reduce the burden on yourself.

When you first begin in private practice, your staff will probably be minimal. Employing staff usually starts with transferring some of the work to an assistant, locum or prospective partner. The hard work, dedication and efficiency of a happy staff can be one of your most important resources when you are developing your practice.

You may worry about obtaining good staff and delegating responsibility. The problem will be solved if you go about it wisely and do not rush into accepting the first comers.

If you are very busy, a natural anxiety may lead you to take on immediate help, but if the new employees are unsuitable you may find it worse than no help at all.

The efforts and competence of good staff are often undervalued or even ignored. The staff do not own the practice, you do, and their attitudes, expectations and demands will differ from yours in many ways. Employing staff can bring problems—they may be ill or have family troubles. You, as the employer, will be close to the problems, especially in a small practice. You will know your staff personally and feel responsible for them. So select them carefully and look after them well. Consideration and kindness will be well rewarded.

Delegation

By delegating responsibility and authority to your staff, you will relieve yourself of at least some of the work load and the time saved will be cost effective if used wisely. Staff are responsible for the performance of their own duties, and the extent of their authority must be clearly understood by both sides, as any decisions made by staff within their sphere of authority are also your decisions as you are ultimately responsible for the overall running and management of the practice. A degree of supervision may be necessary if you wish them to develop initiative and interest in their work and your practice, but have confidence in them and their professional competence.

They may bring knowledge and expertise you lack which will be beneficial to the practice. Delegation will enable you to spend more time on practice management, education and development.

Finally, the confidence and ability gained by staff is in itself a form of training which may lead to them becoming partners in your practice, succeeding you or setting up for themselves.

Recruitment and advertising

Good staff are essential so you must not be afraid to spend money on recruitment. Where will you find staff? Here are a few suggestions:
1. Advertise in the periodicals and journals of the professional organisation to which you belong. You can also advertise in the local or national press.
2. Telephone your professional organisation and see if there is a list of suitable applicants on its books.
3. Contact local medical groups and local hospitals to find out if anyone is interested in the position.
4. Contact the local employment agency. It can screen and check applicants for you.
5. Contact schools, colleges and polytechnics as a suitable student may be looking for a job in the future.
6. Make enquiries of friends or neighbours. They might know someone suitable.

Do ask yourself before you start recruiting whether you really need to take on a permanent member of staff: it might be better to have agency staff or a locum for a short period until you are certain you really need a full-time member of staff. Employee salaries will add to the general overhead expenses. Clarify for yourself exactly why you need staff, and how much you can afford to pay them.

Job description, analysis and specification

Having analysed exactly what skills and experience you need from a new member of staff, you are now ready to specify the content of the job. A simple example of a standard job description might contain the following:

1. The qualifications, skills and experience required for the practice.
2. The level of responsibility.
3. The type of work you expect the candidate to do.
4. The age of the candidate if applicable.
5. The person to whom he/she will be responsible.
6. The remuneration you expect to pay. This enables applicants to have some idea of their prospective salary. The 'market value' of the job is important, so check the proposed salary with other practitioners.

What each applicant can offer may now be directly related to every itemised requirement. This will make it easier to screen and select your staff more effectively. The applicant can also decide whether he/she may apply with any hope of being successful.

Interviews

You should write to or contact by telephone those applicants who appear promising and arrange an interview. You will not find the perfect candidate. Interviewing is an art which can take years of experience to perfect, and the instinct, flair or hunch in selecting the best person is often a matter of luck or intuition.

It is advisable for you to interview more than once before you make a decision, and if you are in any doubt, ask a member of staff to help you make the final decision.

At the interview, a great deal of knowledge about prospective employees can be obtained. You can judge for yourself their personal appearance, grooming, voice, poise and mannerisms, all of which are important. Many applicants may be nervous. Try and put them at their ease and see if you are going to get on well together. This is essential in a small practice. If you wish to see their work then give them a trial to establish their ability.

There are some key questions you should ask during the interview. These will give you some indication of the candidate's competence and suitability:

1. Why does the applicant want the job in the practice?
2. Why did the applicant leave his/her last job?
3. How many previous jobs has the applicant had? Too many changes without justifiable reasons can be a bad sign.
4. What are the applicant's interests outside work?
5. Which other practitioners are known to the applicant and how well does he/she know them?

6. Is the applicant intending to stay for a reasonable length of time?

Keep the interview as natural as possible and allow time for the applicant to ask you questions. Now is the time for other staff members to meet the candidate. Their impressions may be very valuable when it comes to making the final choice.

Personal qualities

The principal personal qualities the applicant should possess are:

1. *Punctuality.* A reliable time-keeper sets a good example and gains the approval of patients and other members of staff.

2. *A pleasant manner.* This is very important when greeting patients or on the telephone. A cheerful smile and sense of humour are essential.

3. *A sound general education.* A good knowledge of subjects outside the required qualification and a willingness to attend courses to widen ability and skill are important.

4. *Poise.* This includes composure, self-confidence and the ability to work under pressure. If the staff are calm and unflustered with a pleasant manner, it will create a good impression with the patient.

5. *Fluency in speech.* The ability to communicate with others clearly, quickly and intelligently.

6. *Tact is essential.* There will be many occasions on which the qualities of discretion and diplomacy are vital.

7. *Honesty.* You want honest and truthful members of staff.

8. *Health.* Staff must be fit. The continuity of treatment and the smooth running of the practice will be impaired by continual absenteeism.

9. *Loyalty and responsibility.* If a member of staff is loyal and carries out responsibilities effectively, it will be a tremendous contribution to a successful practice.

10. *Initiative, attention to instructions and accuracy.* Staff must be capable of taking the initiative when necessary and concentrating and listening to instructions. Mistakes can be costly.

11. *Neatness.* A tidy neat person is an asset. Scruffy clothes and appearance give a very poor impression. The practice has to be kept tidy and attractive: staff who are careless about their own appearance will not give proper attention to the appearance of the practice.

12. *Interest.* Staff must be interested in their work, or they will not be happy doing it.

You will certainly be fortunate if you find someone with all these attributes, but they are important.

Selection

Ask applicants to send a hand-written reply, a resumé of themselves or a curriculum vitae. You can learn a lot about prospective members of staff from their written applications. It is courteous to send a rejection letter if you do not select someone.

You may find it an advantage to have as your first employee an assistant who can serve as receptionist, secretary, typist and general helper!

Employing relatives

Generally, it is not a good idea to have friends or relatives as members of your staff. However, there are exceptions and in those cases you should take into consideration the following points:
1. Make sure they can do the job required competently.
2. Check that family members' salaries are an allowable business expense.
3. Keep an accurate and stringent record of the time they work for you as this will be needed by the accountant in the same way as for any other employee.
4. Treat a member of your family or a friend as you would treat any other member of staff, otherwise there will be resentment.
5. Attend to family matters outside practice hours.

References

If you do not feel you are a confident judge of character you must ask for references. They should be followed up, but they are not always reliable as they may overstate the capabilities or personal qualities of the individual. However, they will give you some clues and prevent you making a disastrous choice. It is a good idea to contact the previous employer directly on the telephone since he is often more forthcoming and reliable in conversation than by letter.

You will require the following facts:
1. The dates of previous employment.
2. The description of the position held and level of responsibility.
3. What salary was paid?

4. The applicant's ability to co-operate with other members of staff.
5. The health record of the applicant.
6. The reason for leaving.
7. Character strengths and weaknesses.
8. Would the referee re-hire the applicant?

CONTRACT OF EMPLOYMENT

A properly drawn up contract of employment is a sensitive document as it clarifies from the outset what the terms of employment are. It need not be complicated, but should set out the following:
1. The rate of pay and how it is calculated.
2. Whether it is paid weekly or monthly.
3. The normal hours of work, and the terms and conditions relating to them.
4. Holiday entitlement and pay.
5. Provision for sick leave and pay.
6. Pension and pension schemes.
7. Any special rates for overtime or weekend duty.
8. Notice to be given by both parties.
9. Grievance procedures.

This may sound a little formal, especially for a small practice, but it is helpful if terms and conditons agreed verbally at interview are set out in writing. It will prevent arguments or disagreements later about what was actually discussed. Some employees may want more complicated service contracts, but these may be difficult and expensive to break.

Wages and salaries

Find out from other practitioners and hospital administrators the current rate for an assistant, receptionist or secretary. You do not have to pay the top rate: on the other hand, you must pay a reasonable salary. It is unwise to offer too low a wage as good staff are usually worth what they ask for, and they will already know the range of salary which should be offered. You must calculate the hidden extras, e.g. paid holiday time, sick leave, your contributions to the National Insurance scheme and any pension contributions you may be paying for your staff. Salaries are best calculated at hourly rates based on an average working week. This makes it easier to work out pay for part-time staff. There should be additional payments for overtime, weekend working and being on call, if appropriate. A bonus scheme of some sort will encourage initiative and reward the hard work of the staff.

Time off, holidays and sick leave

Most practices provide for paid holidays and sick leave. Three or four weeks' holidays seem to be acceptable, although many practices give more after longer service. Although you may work harder than your staff, you can take a day off whenever you choose. Staff cannot do this without asking, so the offer of an unexpected day off is always welcome and shows consideration and thought which will be appreciated.

It is a normal condition of employment to pay staff when they are sick. A problem may arise if an employee, either through an accident or illness, needs a prolonged period off work. This can be very expensive, as not only will you have to pay his salary, but you may need to take on a temporary member of staff which will result in additional expense. The Employers Liability Act will guide you as to your statutory obligations, but you may wish to be more generous if the employee concerned is particularly valuable or important to you.

Safety at work

Many Acts have been passed to make places of work less hazardous for employees. The Health and Safety at Work Act 1974 is the current Act used in the United Kingdom. This states clearly that every employer has a duty to ensure, so far as is reasonably practical, the health, safety and welfare at work of all employees. Inspectors who oversee the implementations of this Act can call at your practice at any time to see if the law is being enforced, and they have the authority to close the practice if this is not the case. It may seem a labour to read this important Act, but you are obliged to fulfil its conditions.

PRACTICE POLICIES

There will be occasions when some of the points listed below will have to be discussed between employer and employee to improve relationships in the practice:

1. Most importantly, the existence of the practice and the jobs it provides are only secured by good service to the patients.
2. The work must be done properly, whatever the personal inconvenience.
3. There can be no passengers. Everyone must pull his weight if the practice is to be profitable and survive.
4. Confidentiality of the patients must be protected at all times.
5. Initiative, hard work and competence will be rewarded.
6. Practice policy in respect of clothing, jewellery and other personal effects should be respected.

You are the head of the practice. Your staff may not share your values completely and it is often hard to criticise staff, but you know where the practice's best interests lie and it is your responsibility to see your goals and ambitions fulfilled if the practice is to be successful.

Personnel management and training

Dealing with staff may prove more difficult than anything else. You have to be a splendid ambassador and diplomat, as good relationships are essential. Morale will be high if you train staff carefully, consult them frequently and reward them well, do not let work become dull and routine. Training staff is very time-consuming, but it pays dividends and they will respect you for keeping your standards high.

Point out mistakes courteously; find out why they happened to prevent them occurring again.

A weekly or fortnightly staff meeting is very helpful. There are a number of topics you will want to discuss, such as:

1. The individual patients and if they are making progress—if not why not?
   It is sometimes a good idea to ask a different member of staff to see the patient if progress is not being made.
2. Any new proposals you may have, such as taking on a new staff member or buying new equipment.
3. Proposals or suggestions put forward by the staff.
4. Any grievances the staff may have, provided they are aired in the right spirit.

Mutual co-operation must exist and be adhered to if increased efficiency is going to result in a successful practice. Teamwork is essential: individual members of staff should be allowed to express themselves fully: in their turn they should accept constructive criticism and be willing to consider new ideas which will benefit the patients.

Keeping staff

Once you have found good staff there is the more difficult task of keeping them! Some practitioners engage staff on a monthly, three-monthly or six-monthly basis and if they are satisfactory they are offered a permanent position. If you are not sure whether to take on extra staff, then holiday time, when possible candidates can start as locums, is a good probationary period to see if they are suitable.

Replacing staff is costly and disruptive. Advertising, the time spent interviewing, subsequent familiarisation and training are expensive. There is also the danger that the departing staff member may set up a rival practice, or join a nearby partnership and take patients away from your practice. It is always disappointing to lose key staff, especially if they leave for reasons beyond your control, such as marriage or family commitments.

You should introduce incentives, such as:
1. A monthly bonus based on the profits.
2. Fringe benefits, for example, medical insurance, petrol expenses or travelling allowances.
3. Gifts at Christmas.
4. Continuing education by sponsoring payment for post-registration courses.
5. The chance of a partnership, if appropriate.
6. Regular salary increases.

All the little extras are deductable expenses and are well worthwhile to keep your staff happy. Above all, give praise and encouragement when it is deserved.

Promotion

Staff appraisal is essential if you are going to keep those with ability and ambition. You must have clear ideas about training and promotion. You should not promote a member of staff for his loyalty or long service, but for efficiency, competence and professional skills. Promotion may mean a salary increase, greater responsibility or perhaps the opportunity of a partnership.

Discharging staff

You will be very lucky if this never arises. It is always awkward and can be unpleasant. However, if it is necessary, you must do it. The grounds for dismissal should be explained fully to the member of staff. The usual grounds are:
1. Incompetence.
2. Theft or dishonesty.
3. Negligence when treating a patient.
4. Unjustified absenteeism.
5. Unprofessional conduct.
6. Violation of confidential information.

There are also other, less tangible reasons for dismissal, such as dislike leading to incompatibility. People do react to each other differently and clashes of temperament or personality are not uncommon. Lack of interest in work and a negative attitude towards the practice is not unknown, but once identified, it must be discussed, as it will affect both staff and patients.

The Employer's Liability Act outlines the procedure to be followed when an employee is dismissed. It is strongly recommended that you are familiar with the relevant parts of this Act as it is easy to go wrong and you may find yourself in great difficulty if an ex-employee decides to cause trouble. If you are in any doubt as to what you should do, seek advice either from a solicitor who has experience in industrial relations or from your professional organisation. The law relating to employment, conditions of service, and dismissal or redundancy is complicated, and advice must be taken if you are not absolutely certain you are right.

EMERGENCY STAFF

Locums

Holidays and sickness will result in absence of staff. Taking on a locum for a short period will help minimise inconvenience to the patients and maintain continuity of treatment.

Agency staff

There are several commercial agencies specialising in the provision of qualified staff. Specify the skills you require, how long you need the person, the type of practice you have and the hours of work.

Discuss all your requirements fully with the agency so the right person can be selected. It is recommended that you see prospective members of staff to be sure that they are right for the practice. If the agency has done its job properly, they will be. It is a wise precaution to satisfy yourself rather than take someone's word for it.

You will have to pay the agency rates, the employer's part of the National Insurance contribution, plus VAT at the current rate. This makes agency staff seem costly, but not as expensive, in the long term, as having insufficient staff in the practice to cope with the work.

CONSULTANCY

You yourself may be asked to consult at the local hospital. Consultants are normally self-employed and are paid a previously agreed fee for their services. They can be a full partner, a salaried partner of the practice or they can be on the medical advisory board of the hospital, perhaps as a director: the hospital is usually registered as a limited company, thereby giving the consultant the privileges of a director with shares in the company.

A consultancy can be a useful arrangement, as the services,

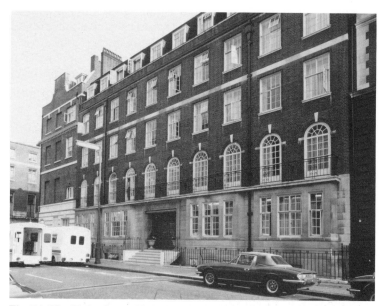

Fig. 7.1 The Harley Street Clinic, London (reproduced by kind permission of American Health Care Ltd).

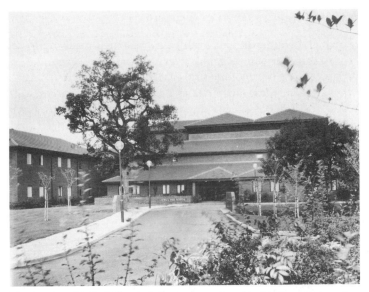

Fig. 7.2 Gatwick Park Hospital, Sussex (reproduced by kind permission of BUPA).

expertise, and maybe a particular specialisation of the consultant will help in building up new referrals and thus enhance the practice, be of benefit to the hospital and improve the general health of the community.

Hospital commissions

If you are asked to see and treat patients in a hospital, there will be several considerations to take into account in order to continue your own practice effectively and successfully and still find time for your hospital patients.

1. You may be asked to visit or treat a patient in a hospital which does not welcome outsiders because it has its own team of medical practitoners. This can be very awkward and you must check with the hospital advisory board in order to establish the admitting rights and whether you will be welcome.
2. You may be asked to treat a patient, and the hospital may then ask you to see other patients on a professional basis; you could also be asked to provide the medical supplies and equipment.
3. The hospital may ask if you would like to rent beds, space and equipment in order to provide services, but otherwise you remain independent.
4. The hospital may wish to employ you full-time.

HOSPITAL PATIENT MANAGEMENT

The growth of independent health care systems, resulting in the advent of more private hospitals every year (Figs. 7.1 and 7.2), is now part of the pattern of medical care in many countries. Finance for these independent hospitals comes from many sources, with industry, medical insurance companies, provident associations and private donations making major contributions.

In answer to the question—why private hospitals when there is a national health care service?—there are a number of benefits to the community of private hospital practice, which are listed below:

1. In rapidly developing areas where accommodation may not be available in an overburdened national health hospital, a patient does not have to wait for admission.
2. There is a choice of the date of admission to the hospital which enables the patient to organise family and working arrangements in time, and the practitioner to arrange his list and scheduling of appointments.
3. Many patients value the privacy of an individual room in which to see the practitioner.
4. There are flexible visiting hours which give the patient's family and friends greater opportunity to see the patient, thereby raising the patient's morale.
5. The patient can have the individual personal attention of the specialist, consultant or practitioner of his choice.
6. There is a choice of facilities in private hospitals which are more accessible.

Private practice and national health care

In the United Kingdom, private beds have always been available in national health care hospitals, although the number has declined. Consultants and practitioners can work full- or part-time for the National Health Service and can admit private patients who pay for their treatment and maintenance.

The advantages and disadvantages have been argued and debated continuously about the existence of a private sector within National Health Service hospitals. Political pressures and government legislation have called for a 'partnership' between the two sectors so that long waiting lists are avoided and expensive equipment is made available to all. Long-term nursing home care is one of the main areas where private facilities are most widely used, thus increasing the availability of National Health Service beds.

Scheduling hospital visits

Proximity to the practice is essential since time spent away from the centre of your work is precious and costly. Travelling is both frustrating and tiring, so only agree to treat or seek a hospital list of patients if it is going to prove worthwhile in the development of your practice.

You must structure your working day by scheduling your hospital visits to fit in with hospital routine, surgical operations, X-rays, meals and baths.

Traditionally, many visiting practitioners see their patients either early in the morning or at the end of the day, but this depends on the nature of the profession. The competition amongst the other professionals to see the patient can be frustrating. Schedule your visit if possible at a time which is not needed by other practitioners. The patient is very often the best guide here.

If you are away from the practice, the time will have to be recovered in respect of fees or a salary, that is, there has to be a return on either your own or the hospital's investment in you.

Admitting rights

Most hospitals have a medical advisory committee or board. You may be invited to take a place on this and certain practitioners will be presented for rights to admit their patients to the hospital. This will be at the discretion of the board. Reputation and word of mouth usually ensures beds for selected practitioners, but if the board and the matron of the hospital do not know you and your work, it will be much more difficult.

HOSPITAL EMPLOYMENT

You may decide to become an employee of one of the independent hospital management groups instead of having your own practice. If so, some factors will apply in the same way as if you were running your own practice, except that you will be responsible for the budgeting, cash flow, development, management and future

forecasting of your services within the group with direct
responsibility to the administrator or the accountants of the
hospital.

Job description

When you first enter private practice, you may have approached the
hospital administrator. He will be anxious to use your services or
perhaps employ you permanently in the hospital. Whichever form
your employment takes, he must give you a joh description and he
will require a curriculum vitae.

Some of the key points to watch for in the terms of the contract
are:
1. Will you be self-employed?
2. Will you bill your own patients or will the hospital send out the
   accounts?
3. Will a consulting room and equipment be provided on a rental
   basis or free of charge?
4. Will you be on a sessional rate at the hospital? Establish sessional
   rates from the professional organisation and other private
   practitioners.
5. What is the insurance cover of the hospital where you and your
   services are concerned? Who is liable?

Interview

You may or may not be interviewed by the hospital administrator
and other members of the staff. They will be looking for high
clinical standards. Although many private hospitals do advertise,
their reputation will rise or fall only on the quality of clinical care
they provide. So if you have a reputation for high standards, hard
work and enthusiasm, you will get the job and the subsequent
referrals.

Do make sure at the outset that your fee or salary is properly
structured so that overtime or on call payments are part of the
standard contract.

The contract

After a successful interview, you should ensure that you receive a
letter of appointment which should set out the following points:
1. The date you are to commence work at the hospital.

2. The fees you will receive if you are being paid as a self-employed consultant or your salary if you are to be an employee.
3. The terms and conditions of the post.
4. A full job description.

There may be a short delay in receiving all the details and the contract, especially if the post is a new one in the hospital. Consult your solicitor if you do not understand the terms of the contract, or there may be an industrial relations section of your professional organisation who will be helpful. Do not sign anything until you are really sure it is what you want and you have checked the contract thoroughly. The law entitles you to certain benefits and the following points may be useful when you are checking a contract:

1. *Pay*
    There should be a statement of the starting salary, and whether it is index linked. There should be details about increments, pay reviews and when you will be paid.
2. *Grade*
    The contract should state your position; for example, will you be the Senior Consultant or an Assistant?
3. *Hours of work*
    These will be given in terms of full- or part-time work. The job may begin part-time and become full-time very quickly, so make sure you have the specific times in your contract which you may have to re-negotiate if this change takes place.
    Do make sure you are paid a fair rate for on call work and that telephone calls are reimbursed.
4. *Location*
    You may have to cover two hospitals for the same hospital group. Do make sure that this is stated and also whether you can claim your travelling expenses.
5. *Holidays*
    The number of days or weeks allowed for annual leave and the number of statutory holidays should be stipulated.
    You may have to be flexible to ensure adequate cover is provided.
6. *Sick leave*
    A reference to any sickness benefit scheme in operation should be included. Private medical insurance companies usually provide good adequate cover within the independent hospital groups.

7. *Period of notice*

   The minimum time that is required to be given by both parties to terminate the contract should be stipulated in the contract.

8. *Pensions*

   As with sickness benefits, the independent hospital groups may use one of the major insurance groups to negotiate the best possible terms for a pension for their staff. All the details should be set out clearly, and the amounts of the contributions and any pension rights if you should change your job must be included. You should ask for a copy of the pension document to show it to your accountant, as he will need it for tax purposes.

9. *Uniform*

   The hospital may have a special style of uniform it would like you to wear which is different from the one you wear in your own practice. Make sure you are provided with an allowance if you have to purchase a uniform.

10. *Equipment*

    If you are taking in equipment from your own practice, do establish who is responsible for maintaining it, insuring it and, most important of all, replacing it. This can be an expensive exercise and electrical equipment especially is often heavy and cumbersome to move. Try and persuade the management to provide what you need at the hospital.

11. There will be details in the contract of how you can pursue a grievance should it become necessary.

12. The Health and Safety at Work Act should be mentioned in the contract and you should make yourself familiar with this Act.

13. *Medical examinations*

    The hospital may ask you to undergo a medical and fitness test before you commence employment. This is understandable for the same reasons as are described in the introduction of this book. The hospital will probably be registered as a limited company and, therefore, seeking to make a profit, they will want fit and able staff.

Informed consent

It is vital that the hospital patient is adequately informed before any treatment is initiated. The implications of this are mentioned in Chapter 4. The same routine must be carried out in the hospital as in your own practice. The patient may be very ill or under the influence of drugs, which may not make him fully coherent about giving consent. Nevertheless, consent must still be obtained before treatment is given. The legal requirements must be strictly adhered to and you should check that the hospital allows you the responsibility of obtaining consent. Certain hospitals only allow their forms to be completed by doctors. There are also specific forms for specific conditions.

Recording hospital patients

You must keep track of your hospital patients. Familiarity with the hospital administration is essential. There may be a card index or computer system kept at the central nursing station. Make sure that all the information required about the patient is fed to this source daily.

You will also need to keep some record back at the practice as there is a strong possibility that the patient may come to you for treatment on an outpatient basis. You will, therefore, require your own notes and records as the hospital records will be retained by the hospital.

Discharging patients from hospital

When a hospital patient is discharged, you will probably have to make a home visit, so allow time to spend with the patient, family and relatives. It is certainly worth it as you will reduce the number of further questions and telephone calls.

General practitioners sometimes outline the four 'D's' to their patients when they are discharged:

1. *Diagnosis*, objectives and prognosis should be explained explicitly in relation to the patient's problem.
2. *Diet* is usually explained as many patients are unsure what and how much they can eat after leaving hospital.
3. *Drugs* or domiciliary treatment may be prescribed. Patients should be cautioned about any side-effects and advised on how to cope with them.
4. *Discharge activity*. Advice must be given about what patients can and cannot do, i.e. when they can return to work, drive a car or play sport. These are all questions patients will want answered when they return home.

Give hospital records a copy of your discharge notes. These should include the following information:

1. The name of the patient.

2. The patient's condition.
3. The hospital reference number.
4. The date of admission.
5. The date of discharge.
6. The referring GP, if any.
7. Clinical history, assessment and treatment.
8. Consultants' names.
9. Any complications.

Follow-up appointments

It is almost a certainty that it will be necessary for you to see your patients at least once after they have been discharged from hospital. They must be given an appointment before leaving the hospital or telephoned immediately they have arrived home. This will preserve continuity of treatment and the patient will feel more secure in the knowledge that you are visiting him at home to ensure he is restored to full health and independence. If another practitioner in the medical team is responsible for the follow-up appointment, make sure full details are given in a clear concise report, with any instructions you would like to be followed for the patient's care.

Hospital patients' accounts

The hospital may be responsible for sending out the patient's account, but if your office has the task, it is necessary to find a system that will keep track of your hospital patients' accounts.

Whatever system you choose, you must ensure that it assists communication between you and your office staff.

There are several systems, such as the following:
1. A card index. This is readily portable and notes can be made on a daily basis whenever you see a patient.
2. A notebook which can be carried in the pocket, recording the full details of the patient. This can be loose-leaf and easily transferred to your own office files when the patient is discharged.
3. A daily list system that is prepared each day and which you give to your secretary or receptionist with the relevant accounting information. This method has the advantage of regular communication between the practice and yourself, and other various activities you may have that day can be added to the list; or if a new patient has to be seen at the hospital, the list can be quickly updated.

N AND HOSPITAL MANAGEMENT 147

PRACTITIONER CHECK LIST

1. Do you really need to take on staff? Will there be enough to keep them busy in six months?
2. Have you worked out a job description?
3. Have you decided how much you can afford to pay?
4. Have you prepared some questions for the interview to determine the suitability of the applicant?
5. Have you taken up and checked references?
6. Have you seen enough applicants for the job?
7. What are the aims of the Health and Safety at Work Act?
8. Have you set out some practice policies for the staff?
9. Have you time for hospital visits?
10. Do you know the legal implications if you are an employee of the hospital?
11. Have you set up a recording and accounting system for hospital patients?
12. Do you wish to seek membership of the local hospital board?

8

Private practice: past, present and future

Historically, private practice is not new. In the United Kingdom, it is only since 1948 that there has been a National Health Service providing medical care for everyone irrespective of his income. Although medicine has been influenced by social, scientific and political changes, the underlying principles of the National Health Service have been the provision of fully-trained, skilled personnel and facilities to provide a service for all those requiring it.

In early civilisations, medical practitioners were paid or punished according to the results of treatment. If it was successful, they were paid an amount related to the social standing or status of the patient. Failure, whether the fault of the practitioner or not, was punished. The severity of the punishment depended on the degree of failure!

The concept of professional standards began with Hippocrates in the 5th century BC. It was further developed in Europe during the Middle Ages by the Church which fostered the provision of medical care through the establishments of the monastic orders specifically to look after the poor and the sick.

The Renaissance saw not only a unique flowering of artistic and creative expression, but also a vigorous intellectual application to scientific and medical matters. The revival of interest in literary, artistic and scientific endeavours, and the emphasis on new learning, led to the development of an attitude and philosophy which centred on human values, and which asserted the dignity and work of man. The Renaissance marked a transitional movement in Europe between medieval and modern times, and its influence lasted into the 17th century.

By the 18th century, raised public expectations of the medical profession and its services exposed the discrepancy between supply and need. An awareness of the appalling medical and social conditions in industrialised and over-crowded urban areas, led to the introduction of the new voluntary hospitals. These provided some comfort and care for those unable to pay for medical help,

148

however badly it was needed. This easily available and free service led the local doctors to feel cheated of their fees. They argued strongly that the patients must come to them first and only be referred to the hospital if it was necessary. The British Medical Association which had been formed in 1856 was very concerned to keep the balance between the now widely accepted necessity of free health care for the 'poor' and a reasonable income for its members.

Despite the enthusiasm, dogged determination and the energy of a few notable Victorian reformers, the 19th century was not renowned for its success in the care of the poor, needy and sick. Victorian attitudes encouraged individual thrift and the concept of making provision against hard times by saving on a regular basis with the new friendly and provident societies. Working men contributed a small amount weekly, making them eligible for medical treatment. This system, however, excluded all those, and there were many, who either had no job, or could not afford the weekly subscription. The schemes, often run by laymen, underpaid and overworked the doctors, so by the early 20th century, it became clear that the interests of both patients and doctors could only be met by some sort of governmental control of supply and demand. Although medical care was still primarily an arrangement between the doctor and the patient on a fee paying basis for those who could afford it, government legislation in the form of the National Insurance Act 1911 began to make inroads into this longstanding and traditional relationship.

The Act of 1911 provided a financial cushion for some members of society in times of illness, and can be seen as the beginnings of a state medical service, whereby there was a shift in emphasis from private control of medical care to state control.

The Second World War brought about changes in public attitudes to state control. The war had necessitated government intervention in all aspects of national life. During the war, through the Emergency Medical Service, all citizens had been given a comprehensive hospital service, and the armed forces had received primary medical care as well. A combination of these two developments provided the foundations of the National Health Service. Whether the hopes, aspirations and ideals which inspired the principles on which the National Health Service in the United Kingdom was founded have been fulfilled, is a matter for both private reflection and public debate.

Today, providing health care for a large population is a multi-faceted problem. The recent rapid growth of private medicine has been in response to a growing desire by patients to exercise freedom of choice.

Private facilities are now more widely available both in geographical and numerical terms, and are no longer confined to the cities and larger towns. In 1979, there were 149 acute private hospitals with just over 6500 beds. By the end of 1984, there were 200 hospitals with a bed availability of approximately 10 000. One of the reasons for this increase is the business activities of companies who have recently joined the ranks of the more traditional providers of health care, the provident societies and the charitable hospitals.

An important result of this development has been the sharp rise in the number of people taking out private medical insurance. It is interesting to note that, at present, many firms are attracted to the idea of offering health care benefits under a group scheme, as part of an employment package. One of the more obvious advantages is that personnel have access to medical facilities at a time and place which is convenient for them and the company, thereby minimising disruption at work.

A very important point which is often overlooked, is that the level of fees charged by the private practitioner is reflected in the premiums paid directly by the patient or his company. Costs, therefore, must be contained or the premiums will escalate to a point beyond the reach of many who now support the private sector.

There are now significantly more practitioners engaged in private work, either full- or part-time, than ten years ago, and this reflects the growth in the insurance market and an increased awareness that private practice offers an attractive employment alternative. Whilst expansion of the private sector has been welcome, there is now sharp competition in this area. Therefore, it is essential for the practitioner to be sensitive to the changing needs of the patient. There is more emphasis on prevention (Fig. 8.1), the promotion of health and the importance of self-care education in the community, so the private practitioner must be flexible as success and future development depend on a swift, vigorous response to market demands.

An almost unlimited range of opportunities exists for the future. Development in areas such as drug abuse, screening and diagnostic services, and initiatives in the care of the elderly and long-stay patients, are now being undertaken in the private sector. Private practitioners should be aware of what is happening in other countries. At world level, health care is enormously expensive, but with the exchange of ideas and greater co-operation, the problems

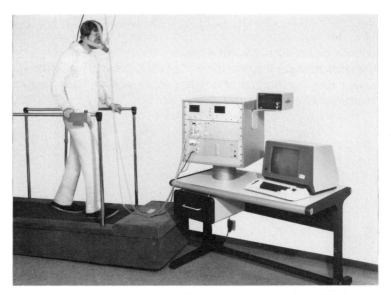

Fig. 8.1 Screening and diagnostic facilities (by kind permission of BUPA).

of health in a world-wide context are being faced internationally. This co-operation will offer greater opportunities for practitioners to participate in these challenging areas of health care and on an international basis.

In the United Kingdom, one of the most important developments already taking place is the increasing degree of co-operation between the private sector and the National Health Service. The sharing of expensive equipment will become more widespread than it is at present, particularly where demand in private medicine is insufficient to justify capital outlay and the National Health Service has the demand, but lacks the funds to buy costly items. Where there are waiting lists in the National Health Service but spare capacity privately, there is a welcome trend for the two sectors to work together in matching supply and demand.

The clinical practitioner working alone, in a small group or in an associate practice, is part of a complex network of national health care provision. The attempts to rationalise and co-ordinate resources may seem far removed from the individual, but the practical applications will deeply affect the way the private practice operates in the future.

Therefore, in order to meet the demands of the future, the private practitioner must be constantly aware of developments in the market place and understand their significance, thereby identifying how his practice must change to meet the challenges the developments will inevitably bring.

Excellent clinical standards and personal care given when and where they are needed at a price which is acceptable, are the cornerstones of a successful private practice.

Bibliography

Barrow C 1984 Financial management for the small business. Kogan Page, London

Bradshaw J 1983 Guide to DIY house buying, selling and conveyancing, 2nd ed. Castle Books, Leamington

Dewis M 1978 The law on health and safety at work. MacDonald and Evans, Plymouth

Elliot A G Your business. The right way to run it. Elliot Right Way Books, Kingswood

Farrell P 1983 How to buy a business. Kogan Page, London

Gaffney M Setting up a new business. HMSO, London

Golzen G 1984 Working for yourself, 7th edn. Kogan Page, London

Knox P 1980 Insurance—are you covered? Oyez and Ward Lock, London

Leigh-Taylor N 1976 Doctors and the law. Oyez Publishing, London

Morris M J 1984 Successful expansion for the small business. Kogan Page, London

Porter D 1976 Profitable management of a solicitor's practice. Oyez Publishing, London

Sinclair W I 1984 Allied Hambro tax guide 1984–1985. Oyez Longman, London

British Medical Association 1981 The handbook of medical ethics. BMA, London

British United Provident Association 1980. A guide to private consultant practice, 3rd edn

General Medical Council 1985 Professional conduct and discipline: fitness to practice

Organisation of Chartered Physiotherapists in Private Practice 1985 Starting in private practice (revised)

Relevant Acts of Parliament

1858 Medical Act
1861 Offence Against the Person Act
1880 Employer's Liability Act
1911 National Insurance Act
1930 Third Parties Act
1946 National Health Service Act
1946 National Insurance Act
1954 Landlord and Tenant Act
1957 Occupier's Liability Act
1960 Professions Supplementary to Medicine Act
1965 National Insurance Act
1969 The Medical Act
1969 Employer's Liability Act
1969 Family Law Reform Act
1970 Administration of Justice Act
1971 Fire Precautions Act
1971 National Insurance Act
1972 Contract of Employments Act
1974 Health and Safety at Work Act
1975 Social Security Act
1975 Employment Protection Act
1976 Town and Country Planning Act
1977 Criminal Law Act
1983 Mental Health Act
1984 Data Protection Act

Appendices

The following appendices give information for the principal countries that are likely to have health professionals wishing to set up in private practice. The countries are listed alphabetically and information for each country has been grouped under the following headings:

Government organisations
Professional organisations
Medical insurance
Taxation offices
Main banks
Private hospitals and clinics
Medical bookshops
Useful sources of information.

The authors have not investigated the organisations listed in the appendices and assume no responsibility for them.

Every effort has been made to ensure the accuracy of the information contained in these appendices and to make them as comprehensive as possible, but there is no responsibility taken by the authors for changes of address, clerical and printers' errors or the exclusion of some bodies. If details can be submitted, future editions can be made more comprehensive.

CONTENTS

Australia, 157
Belgium, 167
Canada, 170
Denmark, 178
Eire, 180
Hong Kong, 183
Japan, 185
The Netherlands, 186
New Zealand, 189
Norway, 191
South Africa, 192
Sweden, 194
Switzerland, 195
United Kingdom, 196
Northern Ireland, 215
United States of America, 216

Australia

Many of the health services are provided on a State basis and, therefore, detailed information must be obtained through the relevant offices. The Yellow Pages of each State will give a lot of information, especially where services are required for the telephone, fire and safety protection and printing.

Government organisations

New South Wales Department of Health
McKell Building
Rawson Place
Sydney 2000
(PO Box K110 Haymarket 2000)
Telephone: (02) 217 6666

Victorian Health Department
555 Collins Street
Melbourne 3000
Telephone: (03) 616 7777

Queensland Department of Health
State Health Building
Brisbane 4000
(GPO Box 48 Brisbane 40001)
Telephone: (07) 224 0545

South Australia Health Commission
158 Rundle Mall
Adelaide 5000
Telephone: (08) 218 3211

Health Department of Western Australia
'Curtin House'
60 Beaufort Street
Perth 6000
Telephone: (09) 328 0241

Tasmanian Department of Health Services
34 Davey Street
Hobart 7000
(GPO Box 191 B Hobart 7001)
Telephone (002) 30 8022

Australian Capital Territory Health
Authority
Moor & Alinga Streets
Canberra City 2601
(GPO Box 825 Canberra 2601)
Telephone: (062) 454111

Northern Territory Department of Health
MLC Building
81 Smith Street
Darwin 5790
(PO Box 1701 Darwin 5794)
Telephone: (089) 802911

Professional organisations

Association of Health Professions
PO Box 162 St Leonards NSW 2065
Telephone: (02) 438 1833 Thursdays only
(02) 389 6425 other days

Association of Medical Superintendents of
NSW & ACT
Campbelltown Hospital
PO Box 149 Campbelltown NSW 2560

Australasian College of Dermatologists
Federal Office
271 Bridge Rd
Glebe NSW 2037
Telephone: (02) 660 5392

Australasian Society of Clinical &
Experimental Pharmacologists
Department of Clinical Pharmacology
Royal North Shore Hospital
St Leonards NSW 2065
Telephone: (02) 438 7631

Australian Association of Clinical
Biochemists
Biochemistry Dept
Royal Perth Hospital WA 6000

Australian Association of Gerontology
Federal Office
Science Centre
35–43 Clarence St
Sydney NSW 2000

Australian Association of Neurologists
c/o Dept Clinical Neuro-Physiology
Alfred Hospital
Commercial Rd
Prahran, Vic 3181

Australian Association of Occupational
Therapists Inc.
PO Box 338 Nedlands WA 6009
Telephone: (09) 380 1122

Australian Association of Social Workers
Federal Office
PO Box 258 Civic Sq.
Canberra ACT 2608
Telephone: (062) 47 3253

Australian Association of Speech & Hearing
212 Clarendon St
East Melbourne 3002
Telephone: (03) 419 0536

Australian Chiropractors Association
8 First St
Murray Bridge, SA 5253

Australian College of Health Service
Administrators
Hornsby & Ku-ring-gai Hospital
Palmerston Rd
Hornsby NSW 2077
Telephone: (02) 476 6148

Australian College of Paediatrics
PO Box 30, Parkville Vic 3052
Telephone: (03) 329 8181

Australian College of Rehabilitation
Medicine
PO Box 341, Ryde NSW 2112
Telephone: (02) 807 6771

Australian Council of Allied Health
Professions
Hospitals Division Health Commission of
Vic
555 Collins St
Melbourne Vic 3000

Australian Council of Social Service
147/149 Castlereagh St
Sydney NSW 2000
(PO Box E158 St James)
Telephone: (02) 290 3466

Australian Dental Association
Federal Office
116 Pacific Hwy
North Sydney NSW 2060
Telephone: (02) 92 0682

Australian Institute of Health Surveyors
PO Box 97 Camperdown NSW 2050
Telephone: (02) 516 2419

Australian Institute of Medical Laboratory
Scientists
National Office
PO Box 450 Toowong Qld 4066

Australian Institute of Radiography
PO Box 278 East Melbourne Vic 3002
Telephone: (03) 419 3336

Australian Medical Association
77–79 Arundel St
Glebe NSW 2037
Telephone: (02) 660 6466

Australian Optometrical Association
204 Drummond St, Carlton Vic 3053
Telephone: (03) 347 0833

Australian Orthopaedic Association
229–231 Macquarie St
Sydney NSW 2000
Telephone: (02) 233 3018

Australian Physiotherapy Association
25–27 Kerr St
Fitzroy Vic 3065
Telephone: (03) 417 5244

Australian Postgraduate Federation in
Medicine
22 Lascelles Ave
Toorak Vic 3142
Telephone: (03) 240 8671

Australian Society for Medical Research
145 Macquarie St
Sydney NSW 2000
Telephone: (02) 27 4461

Canberra & Southern Districts
Pharmacists
PO Box 105 Jamison ACT 2614
Telephone: (062) 51 3220

Capital Territory Group of the Australian
Medical Association
GPO Box 1187 Canberra ACT 2601
Building 4 Woden Valley Hospital
Telephone: (062) 81 2144

Chiropodists Board of Queensland
9th Floor
280 Adelaide St
Brisbane Qld 4000

Clinical Oncological Society of Australia
GPO Box 4708 Sydney NSW 2001
Telephone: (02) 231 3355

College of Nursing Australia
Suite 22
431 St Kilda Rd
Melbourne Vic 3004
Telephone: (03) 266 5145

Dental Board of Queensland
9th Floor
280 Adelaide St
Brisbane Qld 4000

Dieticians Association of Australia
Commercial House
Brisbane & Macquarie Sts
Barton ACT 2600
PO Box E187 Queen Victoria Tce
ACT 2600

Doctors Reform Society (NSW)
L3 243 Cleveland St
Redfern NSW 2016
PO Box 11 Strawberry Hills
NSW 2012
Telephone: (02) 319 1777

Doctors Reform Society (Vic)
PO Box 94 Clifton Hill Vic 3068
Telephone: (03) 481 7544

Doctors Reform Society (Qld)
PO Box 276 Paddington Qld 4064
Telephone: (07) 369 7594

Doctors Reform Society (SA)
GPO Box 946 Adelaide SA 5001
Telephone: (08) 31 3483

Doctors Reform Society (WA)
PO Box 467 Subiaco WA 6008
Telephone: (09) 361 0742

Guild of Dispensing Opticians (Aust) Ltd
12 Thomas St
Chatswood NSW 2067
Telephone: (02) 412 3033

Institute of Nursing Administrators of NSW
& ACT
PO Box 155 Rozelle NSW 2039

Institute of Hospital Engineers (Australia)
PO Box 309 Mt Eliza Vic 3930
Telephone: (03) 528 6333

Medical Administrators of Western Sydney
Campbelltown Hospital
PO Box 149 Campbelltown NSW 2560

Medical Benefits Fund of Australia Ltd
258–262 George St
Sydney NSW 2000
Telephone: (02) 230 9500

Medical Benefits Fund of Australia Ltd
187 Edward St
Brisbane Qld 4000
Telephone: (07) 221 5444

Medical Benefits Fund of Australia Ltd
29 Elizabeth St
Hobart Tas 7000
Telephone: (002) 34 8100

Medical Benefits Fund of Australia Ltd (Inc.
in NSW)
175–177 London Circuit
Canberra City ACT 2601
Telephone: (062) 48 8367

Medical Board of Queensland
9th Floor
280 Adelaide St
Brisbane Qld 4000

Medical Record Association of Australia
GPO Box 4119 Sydney NSW 2001

National Standing Committee of Medical
Superintendents
Manly District Hospital
PO Box 465 Manly NSW 2095

NSW Association of Occupational
Therapists
11 Grose St, Camperdown NSW 2050
Telephone: (02) 51 1006

NSW College of Nursing
55 Hereford St
Glebe NSW 2037
Telephone: (02) 660 7100

NSW Institute of Dietitians
Dept of Dietetics
Royal North Shore Hospital
St Leonards NSW 2065
Telephone: (02) 438 7579

NSW Medical Record Association
GPO Box 4119 Sydney NSW 2001

NSW Nurses' Association
188–192 Goulburn St
Darlinghurst NSW 2010
Telephone: (02) 267 9934

Nurses Board of South Australia
158 Rundle Mall
Adelaide SA 5000
Telephone: (08) 223 4957

Nurses Board of Western Australia
1140 Hay St
West Perth WA 6005
Telephone: (09) 321 3277

Nurses Registration Board of Queensland
9th Floor
280 Adelaide St
Brisbane Qld 4000

Nurses Registration Board of Tasmania
GPO Box 191B Hobart Tas 7001
Telephone: (002) 30 3501

Optometrists Board of Queensland
9th Floor
280 Adelaide St
Brisbane Qld 4000

Pharmaceutical Society of Western Australia
28A Ventnor Ave
West Perth WA 6005
Telephone: (09) 321 4082

Pharmaceutical Society of Australia
PO Box 77 Curtin ACT 2605
Telephone: (062) 81 1366

Pharmacy Board of Queensland
9th Floor
280 Adelaide St
Brisbane Qld 4000
(GPO Box 2438)
Telephone: (07) 227 7111

Pharmacy Board of South Australia
109 Greenhill Rd
Unley SA 5061
Telephone: (08) 272 1211

Pharmacy Board of Victoria
381 Royal Parade
Parkville Vic 3052
Telephone: (03) 387 7222

Pharmacy Guild of Australia
PO Box 36 Deakin ACT 2600
Telephone: (062) 81 0911

Physiotherapists Board of Queensland
9th Floor
280 Adelaide St
Brisbane Qld 4000

Postgraduate Committee in Medicine
Coppleston Institute
University of Sydney
NSW 2006

Postgraduate Medical Education Committee
AMA House, 88 L'Estrange Tce
Kelvin Gve Qld 4059
Telephone: (07) 356 6455

Postgraduate Medical Education Committee
(University of Western Australia)
8 Kings Park Rd
West Perth WA 6000
Telephone: (09) 321 7898

Queensland Bush Nursing Association
National Bank Building
180 Queen St
Brisbane Qld 4000
Telephone: (07) 229 3953

Royal Australasian College of Physicians
145 Macquarie St
Sydney NSW 2000
Telephone: (02) 27 4461

Royal Australasian College of Radiologists
Federal Office
37 Lower Fort St
Millers Point NSW 2000
Telephone: (02) 27 7797

Royal Australasian College of Surgeons
Spring St
Melbourne Vic 3000
Telephone: (03) 662 1033

Royal Australian & New Zealand College of
Psychiatrists
Maudsley House
107 Rathdowne St
Carlton Vic 3053
Telephone: (03) 663 5466

Royal Australian College of General
Practitioners Headquarters
13 Lower Fort St
Sydney NSW 2000
Telephone: (02) 27 3244/8845

The Royal Australian College of Medical
Administrators Federal Office
15 Drummond St
Carlton Vic 3053
Telephone: (03) 663 5347

The Royal Australian College of
Obstretricians & Gynaecologists
254 Albert St
East Melbourne Vic 3002
Telephone: (03) 417 1699

Royal Australian College of
Ophthalmologists
27 Commonwealth St
Sydney NSW 2010
Telephone: (02) 267 7006

Royal Australian Nursing Federation
2nd Floor
132–136 Albert Rd
Sth Melbourne Vic 3205
Telephone: (03) 699 8477

Royal College of Pathologists of Australia
Durham Hall
207 Albion St
Surry Hills NSW 2010
Telephone: (02) 332 4266

Royal District Nursing Society of SA
139 Kensington Rd
Norwood SA 5067
Telephone: (08) 332 6444

Society of Hospital Pharmacists of Australia
PO Box 72 Abbotsford Vic 3067
Telephone: (03) 529 7471

South Australian Postgraduate Medical
Association Inc (SAPMEA)
GPO Box 498 Adelaide SA 5001

Standards Association of Australia
PO Box 458 80 Arthur St
North Sydney NSW 2060
Telephone: (02) 929 6022

Tasmanian Association of Occupational
Therapists
Occupational Therapy Dept
Douglas Palmer Rehabilitation Centre
Tower Rd
Newton Tas 7008
Telephone: (002) 38 1816

Tasmanian Postgraduate Committee in
Medicine
AMA House
2 Gore St
South Hobart Tas 7000

Victorian Association of
Occupational Therapists
24 Golf Rd
Sth Oakleigh Vic 3000
Telephone: (03) 579 1802

Victorian Bush Nursing Association (INC)
130 Lt Collins St
Melbourne Vic 3000
Telephone: (03) 63 6887

Victorian College of Pharmacy Ltd
381 Royal Parade
Parkville Vic 3052
Telephone: (03) 387 7222

Victorian Council of Social Service
292 Wellington St
Collingwood Vic 3066
Telephone: (03) 419 3555

Victorian Medical Postgraduate Foundation
22 Lascelles Ave
Toorak Vic 3142
Telephone: (03) 240 8671

Victorian Medical Record Association
PO Box 12
North Melbourne Vic 3051

Victorian Nursing Council
555 Collins St
Melbourne Vic 3000
Telephone: (03) 616 7777

Medical insurance: companies and national organisations

The Health Insurance Commission, a stationary body, operates Medibank Private, Australia's only national private health insurance fund.

Health Insurance Commission
Medibank House
Bowes Place
Phillip ACT 2606
(PO Box 40 Woden ACT 2606)
Telephone: (062) 83 5411

State offices

Sydney
17 Castlereagh St
Sydney NSW 2000
(GPO Box 9999 Sydney NSW 2001)
Telephone: (02) 237 6222

Melbourne
460 Bourke St
Melbourne Vic 3000
(GPO Box 9999 Melbourne Vic 3001)
Telephone: (03) 607 9222

Brisbane
82 Ann St
Brisbane Qld 4000
(GPO Box 9999 Brisbane Qld 4001)
Telephone: (07) 228 5211

Adelaide
209 Greenhill Rd
Eastwood SA 5063
(GPO Box 9999 Adelaide SA 5001)
Telephone: (08) 274 6611

Perth
50 William St
Perth WA 6000
(GPO Box 9999 Perth WA 6001)
Telephone: (09) 322 1133

Hobart
77 Collins St
Hobart Tas 7000
(GPO Box 9999 Hobart Tas 7001)
Telephone: (002) 34 7999

Registered health benefits organisations

New South Wales
AMA Health Fund Ltd
33 Atchinson St
St Leonards NSW 2065

Cessnock District Hospital Contribution
Fund
View St
Cessnock NSW 2325
(PO Box 154)

The Commercial Banking Co Health Society
343 George St
Sydney NSW 2000
(GPO Box 2720)

Commonwealth Bank Health Society
Pitt St/Martin Place
Sydney NSW 2000
(GPO Box 2719)

The Great United Order of Odd Fellows
Friendly Society of New South Wales
147–149 Castlereagh St
Sydney NSW 2000
(GPO Box 1507)

Government Employees Medical and
Hospital Club
85–87 Smith St
Wollongong NSW 2500
(PO Box 1730)

Health Insurance Commission
17 Castlereagh St
Sydney NSW 2000
(GPO Box 9999)

The Hospitals Contribution Fund of
Australia
403 George St
Sydney NSW 2001
(PO Box 4242)

Independent Order of Odd Fellows of the
State of New South Wales
123 Clarence St
Sydney NSW 2000
(GPO Box 3902)

The Lysaght Hospital & Medical Club
PO Box 77 Port Kembla NSW 2505

The Manchester Unity Independent Order
of Odd Fellows Friendly Society in New
South Wales
307 Pitt St
Sydney NSW 2000

Medical Benefits Funds of Australia Limited
258–262 George St
Sydney NSW 2000

New South Wales Teachers Federation
Health Society
300 Sussex St
Sydney NSW 2000

NIS Health Funds Limited
366 Hunter St
Newcastle NSW 2300
(PO Box 5196C)

NSW Railways & Transport Employees
Hospital Fund
PO Box 2 Petersham NSW 2049

The Phoenix Welfare Association Limited
Industrial Dve
Mayfield NSW 2304
(PO Box 156B Newcastle NSW 2300)

Reserve Bank Health Society
64 Martin Pl
Sydney NSW 2000
(GPO Box 3947)

The Sydney Morning Herald Hospital Fund
Jones St
Broadway NSW 2007
(GPO Box 506 Sydney NSW 2001)

The United Ancient Order of Druids
Registered Friendly Society
Grand Lodge of New South Wales
Druids House
302 Pitt St
Sydney NSW 2000
(PO Box A69 Sydney South NSW 2000)

Western District Health Fund Ltd
Railway Pde
Lithgow NSW 2790
(PO Box 235)

The Wollongong Hospital and Medical
Benefits Contribution Fund
65 Kembia St
Wollongong NSW 2500

Victoria
The Ancient Order of Foresters in Victoria
Friendly Society
55–57 Elizabeth St
Melbourne Vic 3000

Army Health Benefits Society
25–27 Dorcas St
South Melbourne Vic 3205

Australian Natives Association
114–124 Albert Rd
South Melbourne Vic 3205

Cheetham Hospital Benefits Fund
PO Box 272 Geelong Vic 3220

Geelong Medical & Hospital Benefits
Association Limited
60–68 Moorabool St
Geelong Vic 3220
(PO Box 15)

Grand United Hospital Benefit Society
Incorporating the Grand United Order of
Oddfellows in Victorian Friendly Society
140 Bourke St
Melbourne Vic 3000
(GPO Box 633E)

Health Insurance Commission
460 Bourke St
Melbourne Vic 3000
(GPO Box 9999)

The Hospital Benefits Association Ltd
620 Bourke St
Melbourne Vic 3000

Independent Order of Odd Fellows of
Victoria
380 Russell St
Melbourne Vic 3000

Independent Order of Rechabites Friendly
Society
47 Wellington St
Windsor Vic 3181

Latrobe Valley Hospitals and Health
Services Association
32 McDonald St
Morwell Vic 3840
(PO Box 41)

The Manchester Unity Independent Order
of Odd Fellows in Victoria
Manchester Unity Bldg
105 Swanston St
Melbourne Vic 3000

The Mildura District Hospital & Medical
Fund
79 Deakin Ave
Mildura Vic 3500
(PO Box 546)

Naval Health Benefits Society
Room 108 Block D
Victoria Barracks
Melbourne Vic 3004

The Order of the Sons of Temperance
National Division Friendly Society
47–49 A'Becket St
Melbourne Vic 3000

The Protestant Alliance Friendly Society of
Australasia
Grand Council of Victoria
373 Lonsdale St
Melbourne Vic 3001
(GPO Box 5471CC)

Tramways Benefit Society
5 Studley Ave
Kew Vic 3101
(PO Box 207)

Total Care Health Insurance
140 Bourke St
Melbourne

United Ancient Order of Druids
Druids House
407–409 Swanston St
Melbourne Vic 3000

The Victorian District Independent Order of
Rechabites Friendly Society
47 Wellington St
Windsor Vic 3181

The Yallourn Medical and Hospital Society
34 Darilmuria Ave
Newborough Vic 3828
(PO Box 105)

Queensland
Commonwealth Public Service Health
Benefits Society
6 Credit Union Centre
Queen St
Brisbane Qld 4000
(PO Box 1946)

Health Insurance Commission
Medibank Hse
82 Ann St
Brisbane Qld 4000
(PO Box 9999)

Medical Benefits Fund of Australia Limited
Edward St
Brisbane Qld 4000

Professional & Technical Officers Health
Society
Queen St
Brisbane Qld 4000
(PO Box 2384)

Queensland Teachers Union Health Society
St Pauls Tce
Spring Hill Qld 4000
(PO Box 265 Fortitude Valley
Qld 4006)

South Australia
The Advertiser Provident Society
GPO Box 339 Adelaide SA 5001

Health Insurance Commission
209 Greenhill Rd
Eastwood SA 5063
(GPO Box 9999 Adelaide SA 5001)

The Albert District No 83
Independent Order of Rechabites Salford
Unity
2nd Floor ESMA House
52 Gawler Pl
Adelaide SA 5000
(GPO Box 480D)

Mutual Health Association Limited
41 Rundle Mall
Adelaide SA 5000
(GPO Box 990)

National Health Services Association of
South Australia
10 Dequetteville Tce
Kent Town SA 5067

SA Police Department Employees Hospital
Fund
C/o Police Headquarters
1 Angus St
Adelaide SA 5000

SA Public Service Association Health
Benefits Fund
PSA Building
82 Gilbert St
Adelaide SA 5000

Western Australia
Goldfields Medical Fund (Incorporated)
Egan & Cassidy Sts
Kalgoorlie WA 6430
(PO Box 513)

Health Insurance Commission
50 William St
WA 6000
(GPO Box 9999)

Health Insurance Fund of WA
60–62 Stirling St
Perth WA 6001
(PO Box X2221 GPO)

The Hospital Benefit Fund of Western
Australia Inc.
Murray & Pier Sts
Perth WA 6001
(GPO Box C101)

Tasmania
Associated Pulp and Paper Makers Council
Medical Benefits Fund/Hospital Benefits
Fund
Marine Tce, Burnie Tas 7320
(PO Box 201)

Coats Patons Employees Mutual Benefit
Society and Hospital and Medical Benefit
Association
Glen Dhu Mills
Launceston Tas 7250
(PO Box 298)

Health Insurance Commission
77 Collins St
Hobart Tas 7000
(GPO Box 9999)

Medical Benefits Fund of Australia Limited
29 Elizabeth St
Hobart Tas 7000

Queenstown Medical Union Ancillary
Medical Benefits Fund/Hospital Benefits
Fund
Cutten St
Queenstown Tas 7467
(PO Box 294)

Rosebery Medical & Medical Ancillary
Benefits Society
Agnes St
Rosebery Tas 7470
(PO Box 117)

St Luke's Medical & Hospital Benefits
Association
3 The Quadrant
Launceston Tas 7250
(PO Box 915J)

*Professional indemnity insurance for
practitioners*

Medical insurance

Medical Protection Society
165 Bouverie St
Carlton 348 1859

Taxation offices

Australian Taxation Office, PO Box 9990, in
each city in which an office is located.
Principal offices are located in all capital
cities and in Parramatta, Newcastle, Albury,
Dandenong and Townsville.

Main banks

Royal Bank of Australia
ANZ Bank
Westpac Bank
CBA Bank

Private hospitals and clinics

Associated Private Hospitals of WA
7 Shannon St
Floreat Park WA 6014
Telephone: (09) 322 4377

Australian Hospital Association
42 Thesiger Circuit
Deakin ACT 2600
PO Box 344 Kingston ACT 2604

Australian Hospital Association Reference
Centre
Biomedical Library
Monash University
Wellington Rd
Clayton Vic 3168
Telephone: (03) 541 3768/3765/3770

Australian Nursing Homes Association
95–99 York St
Sydney NSW 2000
PO Box Q216 Queen Victoria Bldg
Sydney SW 2000
Telephone: (02) 290 3844

Australian Private Hospitals Association
95–99 York St
Sydney NSW 2000
PO Box Q216 Queen Victoria Bldg
Sydney NSW 2000
Telephone: (02) 290 3844

Hospital Administrative Officers Association
of Victoria
221 Moor St, Fitzroy
PO Box 212 Collingwood Vic 3066
Telephone: (03) 419 0420

Hospital Benefit Fund of WA
125 Murray St
Perth WA 6000
Telephone: (09) 325 9011

Hospital Benefits Association Ltd
620 Bourke St
Melbourne Vic 3000
Telephone: (03) 609 9111

Hospitals & Health Services Association of
New South Wales
1/3 Wharf Rd
Leichhardt 2040
Telephone: (02) 818 3344

Hospitals Contribution Fund of Australia
399–411 George St
Sydney NSW 2000
Telephone: (02) 290 0444

Private Geriatric Hospitals Association of
Victoria
6 Graham Place
Hawthorn East Vic 31
Telephone: (03) 82 1287

Private Hospitals & Nursing Homes
Association of Australia Ltd
95–99 York St
Sydney NSW 2000
(PO Box Q216 Queen Victoria Bldgs
NSW 2000)
Telephone: (02) 290 3844

Private Hospitals Association of Victoria Inc.
The Victorian Chamber of Manufacturers
170 St Kilda Rd
Melbourne Vic 3001
GPO Box 1469-N
Melbourne Vic 3001
Telephone: (03) 698 4111

Private Hospitals Association of Western
Australia
7 Shannon St
Floreat Park WA 6014
Telephone: (09) 322 4377

Private Nursing Homes Association of South
Australia Inc.
Norwood SA 5067
PO Box 633
Telephone: (08) 42 6629

South Australian Hospitals Association Inc.
77 Grenfell St
Adelaide SA 5000
Telephone: (08) 223 1443

Victorian Hospitals Association Ltd
4th Floor
464 St Kilda Rd
Melbourne Vic 3004
PO Box 4360 Melbourne Vic 3001
Telephone: (03) 266 3691

Medical bookshops

Baldings Book Supplies
50 Edencourt Street
Camp Hill
Queensland 4152

CIG Medishield
202 Berkeley Street
Carlton
Victoria 3053

CIG Medishield
103 Rundle Street
Kent Town
South Australia 5067

CIG Medishield
594 Hay Street
Jolimont
Western Australia 6014

Howden Medical
344 Victoria Street
Darlinghurst
NSW 2010

Surgimed Products Pty Ltd
17 Brisbane Street
Hobart
Tasmania 7000

Useful sources of information

Community care

Australian Association for the Welfare of
Children in Hospital
80 Phillip St
Parramatta NSW 2150
Telephone: (02) 635 4785

Asthma Foundation of SA Inc.
Epworth Bldg
33 Pirie St
Adelaide SA 5000
Telephone: (08) 51 4272

Audiological Society of Australia
NAL 5 Hickson Rd
Millers Point
Sydney NSW 2000
Telephone: (02) 20 537

Australian Society of Blood Transfusion
WA Blood Transfusion Service
290 Wellington St
Perth WA 6000

Australian Cancer Society Inc.
GPO Box 4708
Sydney NSW 2001
Telephone: (02) 231 3355

Australian Catholic Health Care Association
1/100 Grey St
East Melbourne Vic 3002
PO Box 73 E. Melbourne
Telephone: (03) 419 9633

Australian Rheumatism Association
Suite 17
Private Consulting Rooms
Royal Melbourne Hospital
Parkville Vic 3050
Telephone: (03) 347 9860

Australian Script for Immunology
Clinical Immunology Research Unit
Princess Margaret Hospital
PO Box 0818
Perth WA 6001

Cardiac Society of Australia & New Zealand
145 Macquarie St
Sydney NSW 2000
Telephone: (02) 27 4461

Community Systems Foundation
A/ASIA
PO Box 605 Crows Nest NSW 2065
Telephone: (02) 438 2233

Gastroenterological Society of Australia
GSA 145 Macquarie St
Sydney NSW 2000
Telephone: (02) 27 4461

Haematology Society of Australia
145 Macquarie St
Sydney NSW 2000
Telephone: (02) 27 4461

The Institution of Bio-Medical Engineering
(Australia)
2 Bridle St
Mansfield Qld 4122

Mental Health Associations
Australian National Association for Mental
Health
23/20 Commercial Rd
Melbourne Vic 3004
Telephone: (03) 26 1938

Neurosurgical Society of Australia
Royal Adelaide Hospital
Adelaide SA 5000
Telephone: (08) 224 5322

New South Wales Council on the Ageing
34 Argyle Place
Millers Point NSW 2000
Telephone: (02) 27 4857

Hosplan (NSW Hospital Planning Advisory Centre)
Kirkbridge 1 Rozelle Hospital
Balmain Rd
Lilyfield 2040
Pvt. Bag 5 Rozelle NSW 2039
Telephone: (02) 818 2922

Technical Aid to the Disabled
PO Box 108 Ryde NSW 2112
Telephone: (02) 808 2022

Thoracic Society of Australia
145 Macquarie St
Sydney NSW 2000
Telephone: (02) 27 4461

Social welfare services

Australian Council of Social Service
147–149 Castlereagh St
Sydney NSW 2000
(PO Box E158 St James, Sydney)
Telephone: (02) 264 8188

Social service agencies and directories

New South Wales
Council of Social Service of New South Wales
34 Liverpool St
Sydney NSW 2000
Telephone: (02) 267 2822

Victoria
Victorian Council of Social Service
290–292 Wellington St
Collingwood Vic 3066
Telephone: (03) 419 3555

Queensland
Queensland Council of Social Service
97 Wickham St
Fortitude Valley Qld 4006
(PO Box 15 Broadway 4000)
Telephone: (07) 52 8544

South Australia
South Australian Council of Social Service Inc
194 Morphett St
Adelaide SA 5000
Telephone: (08) 51 6056

Directory of Social Welfare Resources, South Australia
11th ed. 1985
Published by
Community Information Support Service of SA
84 Franklin St
Adelaide SA 5000
Telephone: (08) 212 4055

Western Australia
Council of Social Service of Western Australia Inc
11 Freedman Rd
Mt Lawley WA 6050
Telephone: (09) 271 0903

Tasmania
Council of Social Service of Tasmania
138 Collins St
Hobart Tas 7000
Telephone: (002) 23 7325

Australian Capital Territory
Directory of Social Services in the ACT
8th edn 1983
Published by
Council of Social Services of the ACT
Griffen Centre
Room 7,
Bunda St
Canberra City 2601
Telephone: (062) 48 7566

Directory of Services for the Ageing
5th Ed 1984 Sept
Published by
ACT Council on the Ageing
Hughes Community Centre
Wisdom St
Hughes ACT 2605

ACT Help Book
Dept of Social Security
Central Administration
Juliana House Bowes Street
Phillip ACT 2606
Telephone: (062) 89 1444

Northern Territory
Director of Community Services in Northern Territory
Published by
NT Council of Social Service
PO Box 5360 Darwin NT 5794
Telephone: (089) 81 8444 or 81 8162

Directory of Services for Older People
The Northern Territory
Published by
NT Council on the Ageing
PO Box 2476 Darwin NT 5794
Telephone: (089) 81 9691

Belgium

In Belgium everyone is obliged to join one of the sickness funds or mutalities. The hospitals have their own medical staff and services while the clinics are private and generally do not maintain resident staff, thus the patient chooses his own physician. Medical practitioners are listed in the telephone book under Liberal Professions, and medical centres, clinics and hospitals are listed in the appropriate sections of Yellow Pages.

Governmental organisations

Ministry of Public Health and Environment
Cité administrative de l'Etat
Quartier de l'Esplanade
B–1010 Bruxelles
Service 'Art de Guérir'
Telephone: 02/564 80 11
Service 'Administration de l'Hygiène Publique'
Telephone: 02/564 80 15
Service 'Inspection Médicale Scolaire'
Telephone: 02/219 44 40

National Council for Scientific Research
8 Rue de la Science
B–1040 Bruxelles
Telephone: 02/511 59 85

Medical Order
Conseil National de l'Ordre des Médecins
32 Place de Jamblinne de Meux
B–1040 Bruxelles
Telephone: 02/736 50 15

Unions of Medical Practitioners
Chambre Syndicale des Médecins de l'Agglomération bruxelloise
13 Avenue de la Couronne
B–1050 Bruxelles
Telephone: 02/649 80 40

Algemeen Syndikaat der Geneesheren van Belgie
34 Sanderusstraat
B–2000 Antwerpen
Telephone: 03/237 32 00

Professional organisations

Groupement Belge des Médecins Spécialistes (G.B.S.)
20 Avenue de la Couronne
B–1050 Bruxelles
Telephone: 02/649 21 47

Groupement Belge des Omnipraticiens (G.B.O.)
76 Rue du Tabellion
B–1050 Bruxelles
Telephone: 02/538 73 65

Société Scientifique de Médecine Générale
Rue de Liège
B–5370 Havelange

Académie Royale de Médecine de Belgique
Palais des Académies
1 Rue Ducale
B–1000 Bruxelles
Telephone: 02/513 26 06
          02/511 24 71

Groupe d'Etudes pour une Réforme de la Médecine (GERM)
29 rue du Gouvernement Provisoire
B–1000 Bruxelles
Telephone: 02/219 67 66

Groupe Médical Cinquantenaire
64 Avenue Albert-Elisabeth
B–1200 Bruxelles
Telephone: 02/735 60 84

Faculteit der Geneeskunde
Secretariaat
Minderbroederstraat 17
B–3000 Leuven
Telephone: 016/22 84 21
Ext: 2577

Universiteitsklinieken St Pieter
Brusselsestraat 69
B–3000 Leuven
Telephone: 016/22 31 01

Universiteitsklinieken St Rafael
37 Kapucinenvoer
B–3000 Leuven
Telephone: 016/22 84 21

Faculte Notre-Dame de la Paix, Namur
Faculté de Médecine
4 Rue Joseph Grafé
B–5000 Namur
Telephone: 081/22 90 61

Rijksuniversitair Centrum Antwerpen
Faculteit Geneeskunde
Universiteitsplein 1
B–2610 Wilrijk
Telephone: 03/828 25 28

Société Royale Belge de Médecine Dentaire
165 Avenue de Jette
1090 Bruxelles
Telephone: 02/426 0347

Sociéte Internationale de Chirurgie,
Orthopédie et Traumatologie
43 Rue Champs Elysées
1050 Bruxelles
Telephone: 02/648 6823

Fédération Médicale Homéopathique Belge
asbl.
59 Chaussée Wavre
1050 Bruxelles
Telephone: 02/511 05 09

Union Professionnelle des Bandagistes &
Orthopédistes de Belgique
189 dr. de Rivieren
1080 Bruxelles
Telephone: 02/425 5561

Union Professionnelle Biologistes
Pharmaciens
4 Avenue Géo Bernier
1050 Bruxelles
Telephone: 02/640 83 70

Société Belge d'Osthéopathie
194b Avenue Tervueren
1150 Bruxelles
Telephone: 02/771 4658

Association des Kinesithérapeutes de
Belgique
29a Avenue A. Buyl
1050 Bruxelles
Telephone: 02/640 4777

Association Professionnelle des Opticiens de
Belgique
26 Rue C. Crespel
1050 Bruxelles
Telephone: 02/512 5526

Groupement des Laboratoires
Internationaux de recherche et d'Industrie
du Médicament (L.I.M.)
49 Square Marie-Louise
1040 Bruxelles
Telephone: 02/230 4090

Association Pharmaceutique Belge & Service
de Controle des Médicaments
137 Rue Stévin
1040 Bruxelles
Telephone: 02/230 2685

Association Générale de l'Industrie du
Médicament (A.G.I.M.)
49 Square Marie-Louise
1040 Bruxelles
Telephone: 230 4090

Main banks

Société Générale de Banque
3 Rue Montagne du Parc
1000 Bruxelles
Telephone: 02/516 21 11

Banque Bruxelles Lambert s.a.
24 Avenue Marnix
1050 Bruxelles
Telephone: 02/517 21 11

Kredietbank n.v.
7 Arendbergstraat
1000 Bruxelles
Telephone: 02/517 41 11

Banque Paris & Pays-Bas
World Trade Centre
162 Boulevard E. Jacqmain
1000 Bruxelles
Telephone: 02/219 30 10

Chemical International Finance &
Consulting s.a.
46 Avenue des Arts
1040 Bruxelles
Telephone: 02/513 54 75

Banque de Commerce s.a.
51/52 Avenue des Arts
1040 Bruxelles
Telephone: 02/513 68 90

International Westminster Bank Ltd.
2–4 Treurenberg
1000 Bruxelles
Telephone: 02/219 40 66

Citibank Belgium s.a.
249 Avenue de Tervueren
1150 Bruxelles
Telephone: 02/761 12 11

Crédit Général s.a. de Banque
8 Rue du Midi
1000 Bruxelles
Telephone: 02/516 12 11

Crédit Communal
44 Boulevard Pachéco
1000 Bruxelles
Telephone: 02/214 41 11

Medical bookshop

Fonteyn Medical Books
Fochplein 13
Louvain

Useful sources of information

Consumer's Association
Association des Consommateurs
Rue de Hollands 13
1060 Bruxelles
Verbruikersunie
Hollandstrat 13
1060 Brussels

National Employment, Information and
Documentation Office
Rue Montoyer 3
Montoyerstraat 3
B–1040 Brussels
Telephone: 02 512 66 88

X-ray

Techniray—X-ray
49 J. Thiebonstrasse Zellick
Brussels
Telephone: 0465 45 79

Medical Personnel

Belgsche Medsche Ketting
Genksesteenweg 1103
Berchem S/A
1080 Brussels
Telephone: 02 466 62 92
             050 60 17 61

Chaine Medicale Belge
1103 Ch. de Gand
108 Brussels

Canada

Canada achieves national health insurance through a series of inter-locking provincial plans which qualify the provinces for federal financial support. The insurance programmes are designed to ensure that there is reasonable access to all medical and hospital care. The protection of the hospital insurance programme is complemented by the Medical Care programme. The advent of the insurance programmes has produced little change in the rights and privileges of private practice. It is advisable to check out the regulations in the province in which you intend to practise. There are government organised local health units and these provide a source of information as well as the Yellow Pages of each province.

Governmental organisations

Department of National Health and Welfare
Ottawa ONK1A OK9
Telephone: 613 990 8188

National Film Board
Box 6100
Stn. A
Montreal QC H3C 3HS
Telephone: 514 333 3333

Department of Veterans Affairs
Veterans Services
Box 7770
Charlottetown PE C1A 8M9
Telephone: 902 566 8888

Statistics Canada
Ottawa ON K1A OT6
Telephone: 613 990 8571

Provincial departments

Alberta
Department of Social Services and
Community Health
10030 107 St
Edmonton AB T5J 3E4
Telephone: 403 427 2734

British Columbia
Ministry of Health
Information Services
Parliament Buildings
Victoria BC V8V 1X4
Telephone: 604 386 3166

Manitoba
Department of Health
Community Health Services Division
831 Portage Avenue
Winnipeg
Telephone: 204 945 6715

New Brunswick
Department of Health
Box 6000
Fredicton NB E3B 5H1
Telephone: 506 453 2536

Newfoundland
Department of Health
Confederation Buildings
Box 4750
St John's A1C 5T7
Telephone: 709 737 3125

Nova Scotia
Department of Health
Box 488
Joseph Howe Buildings
Halifax NS B3J 2R8
Telephone: 902 424 4391

Ontario
Ministry of Health
9th Floor Hepburn Block
Queen's Park
Toronto ON M7A 1S2
Telephone: 416 965 3101

Prince Edward Island
Department of Health and Social Services
Box 2000
Charlottetown PE C1A 7N8
Telephone: 902 892 5471

Quebec
Ministere des Affaires Sociales
1075 Chemin Ste-Foy 2nd floor
Quebec QC G1S 2M1
Telephone: 418 643 6392

Saskatchewan
Department of Health
3475 Albert Street
Regina SK S4S 6X6

Yukon
Health Services Branch
Box 2703
Whitehorse YT Y1A 2C6
Telephone: 403 667 6367

Professional organisations

Academy of Medicine, Ottawa
Box 8223
1867 Alta Vista Dr.
Ottawa ON K1G 3H7
Telephone: (613) 733-2604

Acupuncture Foundation of Canada
7321 Victoria Park Ave.
302, Markham ON L3R 2Z8
Telephone: (416) 474-0383

Association of Allied Health Professionals,
Ontario
2443 Yonge St
Toronto ON M4P 2E7
Telephone: (416) 484-4644

Association des chirurgiens généraux de la
province de Québec
2 Complexe Desjardins
C.P. 216
Succ. Desjardins
Montreal QC H5B 1J8
Telephone: (514) 849-8887

Association of Independent Physicians of
Ontario
2045 Lakeshore Blvd W
Toronto ON M8V 2Z6
Telephone: (416) 259-7034

Association des médecins de langue française
du Canada
1440 Ste-Catherine ouest
#510
Montréal QC H3G 2P9
Telephone: (514) 866-2053

Association des médecins du travail du
Québec
(Occupational medicine)
84 rue de Brésoles
Montréal QC H2Y 1V5
Telephone: (514) 286-1220

L'Association professionelle des
inhalothérapeutes du Québec
(Inhalation therapists)
300 rue Carré St-Louis
#10
Montréal QC H2X 1A5
Telephone: (514) 849-2341

Canadian Anaesthetists' Society
94 Cumberland St
#901
Toronto ON M5R 1A3
Telephone: (416) 923-1449

Canadian Association of
Electroencephalograph Technologists Inc.
Health Sciences Centre
700 William Ave
Winnipeg MB R3E 0Z3
Telephone: 204/787-2836

Canadian Board of Registration of
Electroencephalograph Technologists
(C.B.R.E.T)
The Wellesley Hospital
160 Wellesley St E
Toronto ON M4Y 1J3
Telephone: 416/966-6869

Canadian Association of Emergency
Physicians
c/o Dept of Emergency Services
Sunnybrook Medical Centre
2075 Bayview Ave
Toronto ON M4N 3M5

Canadian Association of Gastroenterology
Jewish General Hospital
3755 Côte Street
St Catherine Road
Montreal QC H3T 1E2

Canadian Association of Internes &
Residents
180 Dundas St W
#1006
Toronto ON M5G 1Z8
Telephone: (416) 979-1182

Canadian Association of Medical Clinics
c/o The Raxlen Clinic
500 Parliament St
Toronto ON M4X 1P4
Telephone: (416) 966-3641

Canadian Association of Medical
Microbiologists
Bacteriology Division
Dept of Laboratory Medicine
Children's Hospital of Eastern Ontario
401 Smyth Rd
Ottawa ON K1H 8L1
Telephone: (613) 737-2543

Canadian Association of Medical Radiation
Technologists
280 Metcalfe St
#410
Ottawa ON K2P 1R7
Telephone: (613) 234-0012
Branches in British Columbia, Alberta,
Manitoba, Saskatchewan, Newfoundland,
Ontario, Quebec, New Brunswick, Nova
Scotia, Prince Edward Island.

Canadian Association of Nuclear Medicine
#806, 1440 St Catherine St
W Montreal QC H3G 1R8
Telephone: (514) 866-2035

Canadian Association of Occupational
Therapists
(Association Canadienne des
Ergotherapeutes)
801 Eglinton Ave W
#401
Toronto ON M5N 1E3
Telephone: (416) 789 2689
There are Provincial Societies in every
province with elected officers. Contact
Toronto address for list.

Canadian Association of Pathologists
4489 Viewmont Ave
Victoria BC V8Z 5K8
Telephone: 604/479-9391

Canadian Association of Physical Medicine
& Rehabilitation
University Hospital (Dept of Rehabilitation
Medicine)
339 Windermere Road
London ON NGA 5AS

The Canadian Association of Radiologists
1440 St Catherine St W
#806
Montreal QC H3G 1R8
Telephone: (514) 866 2035
There are provincial councillors throughout
Canada.

Canadian Athletic Therapists Association
Athletic Injuries Clinic
Humber College
205 Humber College Blvd
Rexdale ON M9W 5L7

Canadian Cardiovascular Society
360 Victoria Ave
#401
Westmount QC H3Z 2N4
Telephone: 514/482-3407

Canadian Chiropractic Association
1900 Bayview Avenue
Toronto
Ontario M4G 3E6

Canadian College of Legal Medicine
#605, 190 St George St
Toronto ON M5R 2N4
Telephone: 416/968-2808

Canadian Council of Blue Cross Plans
c/o 150 Ferrand Dr
Don Mills ON M3C 1H6
Telephone: 416/429-2661

Canadian Dental Association
1815 Alta Vista Drive
Ottawa
Ontario

Canadian Dermatological Association
11 Côte du Palais
Quebec QC G1R 2J6
Telephone: 418/694-5200

Canadian Federation of Biological Societies
Rm 124
118 Veterinary Rd
Saskatoon SK S7N 2R4

Member societies
Pharmacological Society of Canada
Faculty of Pharmaceutical Sciences
University of BC
Vancouver BC V6T 1W5

Canadian Association of Anatomists
Dept of Anatomy
University of Manitoba
730 William Ave
Winnipeg MB R3E 0W3

Canadian Biochemical Society
Dept of Biochemistry
Hospital for Sick Children
555 University Ave
Toronto ON M5G 1X8

Canadian Society for Nutritional Sciences
Dept of Pediatrics
Faculty of Health Sciences
McMaster University
1200 Main St W
Hamilton ON L8N 3Z5

Canadian Society for Cell Biology
Dept of Biology
Laval University
Quebec QC G1V 4G2

Canadian Society for Immunology
Dept of Surgery
Division of Surgical Research
McGill University
740 Dr Penfield Ave
Montreal QC H3A 1A4

Society of Toxicology of Canada/Societe de
Toxicologie du Canada
Box 517
Beaconsfield QC H9W 5V1

Canadian Health Record Association
#301, 1185 Eglinton Ave E
Don Mills ON M3C 3C6
Telephone: (416) 429-5835

Canadian Liver Foundation
42 Charles St E
#510
Toronto ON M4Y 1T4
Telephone: (416) 964-1953

Ontario Foundation for Diseases of the Liver
42 Charles St E
#510
Toronto ON M4Y 1T4

The Canadian Medical Association
Box 8650
Ottawa ON K1G 0G8
Telephone: (613) 731-9331

Provincial divisions
Alberta Medical Association
#304, 9901 108th St
Edmonton AB T5K 1G8
Telephone: (403) 423-2295

British Columbia Medical Association
1807 W 10th Ave
Vancouver BC V6J 2A9
Telephone: (604) 736-5551

Manitoba Medical Association
125 Sherbrook St
Winnipeg MB R3C 2B5
Telephone: (204) 786-7565

New Brunswick Medical Society
#209, 565 Priestman St
Fredericton NB E3B 5X8
Telephone: (506) 454-7745

Newfoundland Medical Association
O'Mara Martin Bldg
135 Military Rd
St John's NF A1C 2E4
Telephone: (709) 726-7424

Medical Society of Nova Scotia
#305, 6080 Young St
Halifax NS B3K 5L2
Telephone: (902) 453-0205

Ontario Medical Association
240 St George St
Toronto ON M5R 2P4
Telephone: (416) 925-3264

Prince Edward Island Medical Society
279 Richmond St
Charlottetown PE C1A 1S7
Telephone: (902) 892-7527

Quebec Medical Association
#1010, 1010 Sherbrooke St W
Montreal QC H3A 2R7
Telephone: (514) 282-1443

Saskatchewan Medical Association
211 Fourth Ave S
Saskatoon SK S7K 1N1
Telephone: (306) 244-2196

Canadian Medical & Biological Engineering
Society
Rm 164
M-50 National Research Council of Canada
Ottawa ON K1A 0R8
Telephone: (613) 993-1686

Canadian Medical Protective Association
Carling Sq, 560 Rochester St
Box 8225
Ottawa ON K1G 3H7
Telephone: (613) 236-2100

Canadian Neurological Society
The Montreal General Hospital
1650 Cedar Ave
Montreal QC H3G 1A4

Canadian Ophthalmological Society
Box 8844
Ottawa ON K1G 3J2
Telephone: (613) 731-6493

Canadian Orthopaedic Association
1117 St Catherine St W
#223
Montreal QC H3B 1H9
Telephone: (514) 844-9818

Canadian Orthoptic Society
Victoria Hospital Corp
375 South St
London ON N5Y 4V3

Canadian Osteopathic Association
575 Waterloo St
London ON N6B 2R2
Telephone: (519) 439-5521

Provincial affiliates
B.C.: Flora Barr, D.O.
461 Martin St
Penticton BC V2A L1
Ont.: Wm. K. Church, D.O.
85 Neywash St
Orillia ON L3V 1X4
Telephone: 705/326-9551
Prairie: Doris M. Tanner, D.O.
2228 Albert St
Regina SK S4P 2V2

Canadian Paediatric Society
Children's Hospital of Eastern Ontario
401 Smyth Rd
Ottawa ON K1H 8L1
Telephone: 613/737-2728

Canadian Physiotherapy Association
44 Eglinton Ave W
#201
Toronto ON M4R 1A1
Telephone: (416) 485-1139
Branches and/or Districts in all provinces.

Canadian Podiatry Association
3414 Dixie Road
401 Mississaga
Ontario L4Y 2B1

Canadian Psychiatric Association
225 Lisgar St
#103
Ottawa ON K2P 0C6
Telephone: (613) 234-2815
Chief Administrative Officer,
Mrs L. C. Metivier

Canadian Psychoanalytic Society (1967) Inc.
7000 Côte des Neiges Rd
Montreal QC H3S 2C1
Telephone: (514) 738-6105

Canadian Speech and Hearing Association
Convention Mezzanire
Royal York Hotel
100 Front Street West
Toronto
Ontario M5T 1E3

Canadian Society of Aviation Medicine
c/o Canadian Aeronautics & Space Institute
#60
75 Sparks St
Ottawa ON K1P 5A5
Telephone: (613) 234-0191

Canadian Society for Clinical Investigation
Laboratory of Molecular Endocrinology
Royal Victoria Hospital
Montreal QC H3A 1A1
Telephone: 514/842-8989

Canadian Society of Cytology
Dept of Pathology
Kingston General Hospital
Kingston ON K7L 2V7

Canadian Society of Laboratory
Technologists
Box 830
Hamilton ON L8N 3N8
Telephone: (416) 528-8642

Canadian Society of Orthopaedic
Technologists
#200, 4433 Sheppard Ave E.
Agincourt ON M1S 1V3
Telephone: (416) 292-0687

Canadian Society of Otolaryngology—Head
& Neck Surgery
c/o McMaster Bldg
170 Elizabeth St
#668
Toronto ON M5G 1E8
Telephone: (416) 598-7102
Secretary, Dr Wm Crysdale
Hospital for Sick Children
Toronto

Canadian Society of Plastic & Reconstructive
Surgeons
#906, 1849 Yonge St
Toronto ON M4S 1Y2

Canadian Society of Respiratory
Technologists
#406, 504 Main St
Winnipeg MB R38 1B8
Telephone: (204) 942-6798
Official journal: 'Respiratory Technology'

Canadian Society for Tropical Medicine &
International Health
1335 Carling Ave
#210
Ottawa ON K1Z 8N8

Canadian Surgical Trade Association
222 Dixon Rd
#305
Weston ON M9P 2M2
Telephone: (416) 243-0524

College of Family Physicians of Canada
4000 Leslie St
Willowdale ON M2K 2R9
Telephone: (416) 493-7513

Corporation professionnelle des
orthophonistes et audiologistes du Quebec
(Speech & Hearing Society)
4770 rue de Salaberry
Montreal QC H4J 1H6
Telephone: (514) 332-9090

Federation of Medical Specialists of Quebec
2 Complexe Desjardins
#3000
Montréal QC H5B 1G8
Telephone: (514) 288-7277

Federation of Medical Women of Canada
#201A, 1815 Alta Vista Dr
Ottawa ON K1G 3Y6
Telephone: (613) 731-1026

Federation des médecins omnipraticiens du
Québec
#1100, 1440 ouest Ste-Catherine
Montreal QC H3G 1R8
Telephone: (514) 878-1911

Federation of Provincial Medical Licensing
Authorities
1867 Alta Vista Dr
Box 8650
Ottawa ON K1G 3H7

Provincial licensing bodies
College of Physicians & Surgeons of Alberta
9901 108 St
Edmonton AB T5K 1G9
Telephone: 403/423-4764

College of Physicians & Surgeons of British
Columbia
1807 W 10th Ave
Vancouver BC V6J 2A9
Telephone: 604/736-5551

College of Physicians & Surgeons of
Manitoba
#1410, 155 Carlton St
Winnipeg MB R3C 3H8
Telephone: 204/947-1694

College of Physicians & Surgeons of New
Brunswick
10 Prince Edward St
Saint John NB E2L 4M5
Telephone: 506/652-5221

Newfoundland Medical Board
15 Rowan St
St John's NF A1B 2X2
Telephone: 709/726-8546

Provincial Medical Board of Nova Scotia
#3050, 1515 South Park St
Halifax NS B3J 2L2
Telephone: 902/422-5823

College of Physicians & Surgeons of Ontario
80 College St
Toronto ON M5G 2E2
Telephone: 416/961-1711

Medical Council of Prince Edward Island
206 Spring Park Rd
Charlottetown PE C1A 3Y9
Telephone: 902/894-5316

Professional Corporation of Physicians of
Quebec/Corporation Professionnelle des
Medecins du Quebec
1440 St Catherine St W
#914
Montreal QC H3G 1S5
Telephone: 514/878-4441

College of Physicians & Surgeons of
Saskatchewan
211 Fourth Ave S
Saskatoon SK S7K 1N1
Telephone: 306/244-7355

The Medical Council of Canada
1867 Alta Vista Dr
Box 8234
Ottawa ON K1G 3H7
Telephone: 613/521-6012

Medical Group Management Association of
Canada
1355 S Colorado Blvd
#900
Denver CO 80222
Telephone: (303) 753 1111

Occupational Medical Association of Canada
c/o Medical Services
7th fl.
290 Yonge St
Toronto ON M5B 1C8
Telephone: 416/591-4242
or at
Box 670
Fenelon Falls ON K0M 1N0
Telephone: 705/887-2532

Ontario Medical Secretaries' Association
240 St George St
Toronto ON M5R 2P4
Telephone: (416) 925-3264

Ontario Psychological Association
1407 Yonge St
#402
Toronto ON M4T 1Y7
Telephone: (416) 961-5552

Royal College of Physicians & Surgeons of
Canada
74 Stanley Ave
Ottawa ON K1M 1P4
Telephone: 613/746-8177

The Society of Obstetricians &
Gynaecologists of Canada
14 Prince Arthur Ave
#210
Toronto ON M5R 1A9
Telephone: (416) 923-3513

Syndicat des Professionnels et des
Techniciens de la Santé du Québec
(S.P.T.S.Q.)
C.P. 2165
St-Romuald QC G6W 5M5
Telephone: (416) 839-5690

Medical insurance

Provincial departments

Alberta
Alberta Dept of Hospitals and Medical Care
Box 2222
11010 101 Street
Edmonton, AB T5J 2P4

2nd Floor
407 8th Ave SW
Calgary AB T2P 1E5

Health Care Insurance Plan
Edmonton
Groat Road & 118th Ave
Box 1360
T5J 2N3
Telephone: 403/427-1432

Calgary
629B 7th Avenue SW
T2P 0Y9
Telephone: 403/261-6411

British Columbia
British Colombia Medical Services
Commission
1515 Blanshard Street
Victoria BC V8W
Telephone: 604/386-3166

Hospital Programs
Ministry of Health
1515 Blanshard Street
Victoria BC V8W 3C8
Telephone: 604/387-1066

Manitoba
Manitoba Health Services Commission
599 Empress Street
Box 925
Winnipeg MB R3C 2T6
Telephone: 204/786-7107

New Brunswick
Hospital/Medicare New Brunswick
Insured Services Division
Department of Health
Box 5100
Fredericton, NB E3B 5G8
Telephone: 506/453-2161

Newfoundland
Newfoundland Medical Care Commission
Elizabeth Towers
Elizabeth Avenue
St John's NF A1C 5J3
Telephone: 709/722-6980

Hospital Services Division
Department of Health
Confederation Building
Box 4750
St John's NF A1C 5T7
Telephone: 709/737-3105

Nova Scotia
Nova Scotia Health Services & Insurance
Commission
Box 760
Halifax NS B3J 2V2
Telephone: 902/424-8902

Ontario
Ontario Health Insurance Plan (OHIP)
Head Office
49 Place d'Armes
2nd Floor
Kingston ON K7L 5J3
Telephone: 416/598-6800

General inquiries should be directed to local
district offices as follows:

Toronto 416/482-1111
Hamilton 416/521-7100
Mississauga 416/275-2730
Oshawa 416/576-2870
London 519/433-4561
Ottawa 613/237-9100
Sudbury 705/675-4245
Kingston 613/546-3811

Thunder Bay 807/475-1423
Special Services Unit
Toronto, 416/965-1000

Prince Edward Island
Prince Edward Island Health Services
Commission
Box 4500
Charlottetown, PE C1A 7P4
Telephone: 902/892-4281

Hospital Services Commission of P.E.I.
Box 4500
Charlottetown, PE C1A 7P4
Telephone: 902/892-4281

Quebec
Regie de l'assurance-maladie du Quebec
(Health Insurance Board)
Box 6600
Quebec QC G1K 7T3
Telephone: 418/643-9407

Hospital Insurance
Ministere des Affaires sociales
1075 Ch. St-Foy
Quebec, QC G1S 2M1
Telephone: 418/643-3005 (est)
and 643-5305 (ouest)

Saskatchewan
Saskatchewan Medical Care Insurance
Commission
3475 Albert Street
Regina, SK S4S 6X6
Telephone: 306/565-3475

Saskatchewan Hospital Services Plan
3475 Albert Street
Regina, SK S4S 6X6
Telephone: 306/565 3269

North West Territories
North West Territories
Health Insurance Admin
N.W.T. Health Care Plan
Government of N.W.T.
Yellowknife NT X1A 2L9
Telephone: 403/873-7714

Yukon
Yukon Health Care Insurance Plan
Box 2703
Whitehorse YT Y1A 2C6
Telephone: 403/667-5367

Yukon Hospital Insurance Services
Box 2703
Whitehorse YT Y1A 2C6
Telephone: 403/667-5233

Other insurance

Blue Cross
150 Ferrand Drive
Don Mills
Ontario M3L 3ES

Blue Cross of Atlantic Canada
PO Box 220
Moncton
New Brunswick E1C 8L3

Cumba Co-operative Health Services
562 Eglington Avenue East
Toronto
Ontario

Hospital Medical Care Plan
710 Bay Street
Toronto
Ontario

Maritime Medical Care Incorporated
5675 Spring Garden Road
Halifax
Nova Scotia B3V 1H2

United Health Services Corporation
Manitoba Blue Cross
100A Polo Park
PO Box 1046
Winnipeg
Manitoba R3C 2X7

Taxation offices

Revenue Canada
Taxation department
55 Bloor Street West
Toronto
Ontario M4W 1A4

Revenue Canada
Taxation department
Ottawa

Main banks

Bank of Alberta
Bank of British Columbia
Bank of Montreal
National Bank of Canada
Bank of Nova Scotia
Royal Bank of Canada
Toronto Dominion Bank
Western and Pacific Bank of Canada

Private independent hospitals and clinics

Ontario Nursing Home Association
6075 Yonge Street
Willowdale
Ontario M2M 3W2

The Canadian Back Clinic
60 Grosvenor Street
Toronto
Ontario M5

Medical bookshops

University of British Columbia Book Store
2075 Westbrook Mall
Vancouver, BC V6T 1W5

University of Calgary Medical Book Store
3330 Hospital Drive N.W.
Health Services Centre
Calgary, Alberta T2N 1N4

University of Alberta Book Store
Students Union Building
88th Avenue–114th Street
Edmonton, Alberta G6G 2J7

McMaster University Medical Book Store
Chedoke-McMaster Hospital
1200 Main Street West
Hamilton, ON L8N 3Z5

University of Toronto Medical Book Store
214 College Street
Toronto, ON M5P 3A1

McGill University Medical Book Store
3655 Drummond Street
Montreal, Quebec
H3G 1Y6

Useful sources of information

The Canadian Arthritis and
Rheumatism Society
Canadian Heart Foundation
Canadian Red Cross

Migraine Foundation
390 Brunswick Avenue
Toronto
Ontario M5R 2Z4
Telephone: 416 920 4916

Multiple Sclerosis Society of Canada
130 Bloor Street West
700 Toronto
Ontario M5S 1N5
Telephone: 416 922 6065

Muscular Dystrophy Association
National Cancer Institute
Order of St John
Victorian Order of Nurses

Telephone sales

Bell Telephone—see the Yellow Pages of the
individual province.

Denmark

Health and medical care in Denmark is financed almost exclusively out of public funds. Health and medicine come under three Ministries. In addition, a National Health Board has the responsibility of advising all public and private institutions in the health field. Although there are opportunities for private practice in Denmark, they are limited.

Government health organisations

National Board of Health
St Kongensade 1
1264 Copenhagen K
Telephone: 01-14 10 11

Ministry of the Interior
Christiansborg Slotsplads
DK 1218 Copenhagen K
Telephone: 01 11 60 00

Professional organisations

Danish Medical Association
Trondhkemsgade 9
2100 Kobenhaven
Telephone: 01-38 55 00

Dansk Tandlaegeforening
Danish Dental Association
Amaliegade 17
Postbox 143
1004 Kobenhaven K

Danske Fysioterapeuter
Norre Voldgade 90
1358 Copenhagen K

The Danish Occupational Therapists
Ergoterapeutforeningen
Nerre Voldgade 90
Postbox 1027
1007 Kobenhaven K
Telephone: 01-13 82 11

University faculties of health

University of Copenhagen
Faculty of Medicine
Panum Institute
Blegdamsvej 3
DK 22 Copenhagen N
Telephone: 01-35 79 00

University of Arhus
Faculty of Medicine
Katrinebjergvej 67, 5
DK-8200 Arhus N
Telephone: 06-16 11 00

University of Odense
Faculty of Medicine
Campusvej 55
DK-5230 Odense M
Telephone: 09-15 86 00

Society for prosthetics and orthotics

International Society for Prosthetics and Orthotics
Borgervaeget 5, DK-2100
Telephone: 00945 1207260

Placement bureaux

Danish Medical Association
Placement Bureau
Tronhjemsgade 9
DK-2100 Copenhagen
Telephone: 01-38 55 00

Bureau of Vacancies
Laegkresdsforeningen for Arhus Amt
Jelshojvej 3
Skade, DO-8270 Hojbjerg
Telephone: 06-27 37 00

Laegekredsforeningen for Fyns Amt
Bureautet
SKt Anne Plads 2–4
5000 Odense
Telephone: 09-13 32 11

Residence and working permits

EC Information Office
St Kongensgade 1
DK-1264 Copenhagen K
Telephone: 01-14 10 11

Directorate for Aliens
Absalonsgade 9
1658 Copenhagen
Telephone: 01-21 11 77

Medical insurance

Laegernes Pensionkasse
Esplanaden BA
DK-1263 Copenhagen K
Telephone: 01-12 21 41

Medical bookshops

Medicinerladen
Norre Alle 32
8000 Aarhus C

Eire

Medical practitioners in Ireland tend to have both public and private patients. About one third of the population is insured with the Voluntary Health Insurance Boards. The VHI operates an insurance scheme which aims to cover the cost of treatment in the private sector.

Government organisations

Department of Health
Custom House
Dublin 1

Health boards

Eastern
Dublin City and County
Kildare and Wicklow
1 James Street
Dublin 8
Telephone: (01) 537951

Midland
Laoighis, Longford
Offaly and Westmeath
Arden Road
Tullamore
Co Offaly
Telephone: 0506 21868

Mid-western
Limerick City and Counties
Clare and Tipperary
31/33 Catherine Street
Limerick
Telephone: 061 316655

North-eastern
Cavan, Louth
Meath and Monaghan
Ceanannus Mor
Co. Meath
Telephone:
Ceanannus Mor 341/046 40341

North-western
Donegal, Leitrim and Sligo
Manorhamilton
Co Leitrim
Telephone:
Manorhamilton 123/072 55123

South-eastern
Waterford City and County
Carlow, Kilkenny, Tipperary and Wexford
Lacken
Dublin Road
Kilkenny
Telephone: 056 21702

Southern
Cork City and County
Kerry
Cork Farm Centre
Dennehy's Cross
Cork
Telephone: 021 45011

Western
Galway, Mayo and Roscommon
Regional Hospital
Merlin Park
Galway
Telephone: 091 51131

Professional organisations

The Medical Council
8 Lower Hatch Street
Dublin 2
Telephone: 0001 602622

Irish Medical Organisation
10 Fitzwilliam Place
Dublin 2
Telephone: 0001 761793

Irish Dental Association
29 Kenilworth Square
Dublin 6

Irish Society of Chartered Physiotherapists
2 Sandymount Green
Dublin 4

Irish Veterinary Association
53 Landsdowne Road
Dublin 4

Medical insurance: companies and national organisations

The Voluntary Health Insurance Board
VHI House
Lower Abbey Street
Dublin 1
Telephone: 01 724499

35/36 Lower Georges Street
Dun Laoghaire
Telephone: 01 800306

VHI House
70 South Mall
Cork
Telephone: 021 504188

Ross House
Victoria Place
Galway
Telephone: 091 63715

62 O'Connell Street
Limerick
Telephone: 061 316122

Taxation offices

Dublin (IT) No 11
4th floor
Setanta Centre
Nassau Street
Dublin 2
Telephone: 71 00 14

PAYE Dublin Districts
Unit nos 710 711 712
3rd floor
Hammam Buildings
11 O'Connell Street
Dublin 1
Telephone: 74 68 21

Hospitals and health boards
580 1st floor
Aras an Phiarsaigh
Pearse Street
Dublin 2
Telephone: 71 53 55

Main banks

Allied Irish Banks
Bank Centre
PO Box 452
Ballsbridge
Dublin 4
Telephone: 600311

Bank of Ireland
Lower Baggot Street
Dublin 2
Telephone: 785744

Northern Bank Ltd
Griffin House
7/8 Wilton Terrace
Dublin 2
Telephone: 785066/766694

Ulster Bank Ltd
College Green
Dublin 2
Telephone: 777623

Private hospitals and clinics

Bon Secours
Glasneirn
Dublin 11

St Vincent's Private Hospital
Herbert Avenue
Dublin 4

Mount Carmel
Braemor Park
Dublin 14

Monkstown Hospital
Monkstown
County Dublin

St Michael's Hospital
Dunlaoghaire
County Dublin

Blackrock Clinic
Blackrock
County Dublin

Medical bookshops

Fannin and Company Ltd
49 Lower Kevin Street
Dublin

Fred Hanna
27/29 Nassau Street
Dublin

Hodges Figgis
56 Dawson Street
Dublin

Surgical Distributors
37 Dawson Street
Dublin

Useful sources of information

Information Section
Department of Health
Room 36A
Custom House
Dublin 1

Social Welfare Department of Disablement
Store Street
Dublin 1
Telephone: 78 64 44

Hong Kong

Government health organisations

Medical and Health Department
10 Hysan Avenue
Sunning Place 9th Floor
Causeway Bay
Telephone: 5-7900896

Health Service Administrators
Prince Philip Dental Hospital
34 Hospital Road
Sai Ying Pun

Community Medicine
c/o Kowloon Regional Office
14th Floor
Golden Gate Commercial Building
136–138 Austin Road
Kowloon
Telephone: 3-721 18953 Ext. 211

Professional organisations

Hong Kong Medical Association
GPO Box 1957
Duke of Windsor Buildings
5th Floor
15 Hennessy Road
Hong Kong
Telephone: 5-278285

Hong Kong Dental Association
Duke of Windsor Social Service Building
8th Floor
15 Hennessy Road
Hong Kong
Telephone: 5-285327

Hong Kong Physiotherapy Association
PO Box 10139
General Post Office
Hong Kong

Hong Kong Chiropractors Association
Room 601
Capitol Centre
5–19 Jardine's Bazaar
Causeway Bay
Hong Kong

Hong Kong Occupational Therapists
Association
PO Box 98241
Tsim Shatsui Post Office
Kowloon

Hong Kong Association of Speech
Therapists
Flat N3
28 Scenic Villas
Victoria Road
Hong Kong

Hong Kong Nurses Association
12th Floor
Hyde Centre
Flat AD
221–226 Gloucester Road
Hong Kong
Telephone: 5-729255

Medical insurance

BUPA Ltd
Room 178
Sun Hung Kai Centre
30 Harbour Road
Wanchai

Private Patients Plan
New World Tower
Central
Hong Kong

Blue Cross (Asia Pacific) Insurance Ltd
2nd Floor
180 Gloucester Road
Wanchai

Medical insurance for practitioners

Medical Protection Society Ltd
c/o The Hong Kong Medical Association
Duke of Windsor Social Service Building
5th Floor
15 Hennessy Road
Hong Kong

Taxation offices

Inland Revenue
Windsor House
311 Gloucester Road
Hong Kong

Main banks

Hong Kong and Shanghai Banking
Corporation
1 Queen's Road Central
Hong Kong

Standard Chartered Bank
4 Des Voeux Road Central
Hong Kong

Private independent hospitals and clinics

Queen Elizabeth Hospital
Gascoigne Road
Kowloon

Princess Margaret Hospital
Lai Chi Kok
Kowloon

Queen Mary Hospital
Pokfulam Road

Princess of Wales Hospital
Shatin
Kowloon

Kisong Wah Hospital
Waterloo Road
Kowloon

Medical bookshops

Swindon Book Co Ltd
13–15 Lock Road
Tsimshatsui
Kowloon

Chung Hwa Book Co Ltd
M/F, 450–452 Nathan Road
Mongkok
Kowloon

Cosmos Books Ltd
30 Johnston Road, Basement
Wanchai
Hong Kong

Man Yuen Book Co
45 Parkes Street
Ground Floor
Kowloon

Times Bookcentre
Shops C & E Milton Mansion
96 Nathan Road
Kowloon

Hong Kong Book Centre
On Lok Yuen Building
25 Des Voeux Road Central
Hong Kong

Commercial Press Co Ltd
9–15 Yee Wo Street
1/F, Causeway Bay
Hong Kong

Joint Publishing Co
9 Queen Victoria Street
Ground Floor, Central
Hong Kong

Sincere Co Ltd
173 Des Voeux Road
Central
Hong Kong

H. W. Chan
PO Box 60023
Tsat Tsz Mui Post Office
Hong Kong

Useful sources of information

Fire and safety

Fire Prevention Services Bureau
1 Asian Buildings
Hennessy Road
Hong Kong

Fire Services Department
323 Java Road
Hong Kong

Telephone sales and directories

GTE Directories (HK) Ltd
23rd Floor
Fortress Towers
King's Road
North Point

Sports organisations

The Sports Club
1–3 Wyndham Street
4th Floor
South China Buildings
Hong Kong

Japan

The opportunities for private practice in Japan are extremely limited, although considerable interest has been shown.

Professional organisations

Japan Association of Occupational
Therapists
2–22–32 Nakamachi
Kogarei-shi
Tokyo

Japan Chiropractors Association
5–9 3-Chome Kita-Aoyama
Minato-kue
Tokyo

Japan Dental Association
3–16 Hayabusa-cho
Chiyoda-kue
Tokyo

Japan Medical Assocation
52-Chome Kanda Surugadai
Chiyoda-kue
Tokyo 101

Japanese Physical Therapy Association
c/o Nimoto Building
2–4–12 Fujami
Chiyoda-kue
Tokyo

Japanese Speech, Language & Hearing
Association
The Research Institute for the Education of
Exceptional Children
Tokyo Gakuoei University
1–1 3-Chome
Nokuikita-machi
Tokyo 184

The Netherlands

Health care facilities are financed mainly through the government insurance system. However, many people in higher income ranges are able to take out private health insurance thereby covering any exceptional medical expenses.

Governmental organisations

National Institute of Health and
Environmental Protection
Postbus 1
3720 BA Bilthoven
Telephone: 030-749111

State Institute for Drug Control
Willem Barentzstraat 7
2315 TZ Leiden
Telephone: 071-121145

National Advisory Council for Public Health
Postbus 7100
2701 AC Zoetermeer
Telephone: 079-517644

Health Council
Postbus 95379
2509 CJ The Hague
Telephone: 070-471441

Health Insurance Funds Council
Postbus 396
1180 BD Amstelveen
Telephone: 020-434747

Hospitals Council
Churchilllaan 11
3527 GV Utrecht
Telephone: 030-739911

Central Council for Health Care Charges
Postbus 3017
3502 GA Utrecht
Telephone: 030-910383

Professional organisations

The Netherlands Medical Association
Koninklijke Nederlansche Maatschappij tot
Bevprderomg Der Geneeslimst
Lomanlann 103
Postbus 20051
3502 LB Utrecht

Dutch Dental Association
Geelgors 1
PO Box 2000
3430 CA Nieuwegein

Nederlands Genootschap voor
Physiotherapie
Van Hogendorplan 8
PO Box 248
3800 AE Amersfoort
Telephone: 033-622400

Nederlandse Bereniging voor Ergotherapie
Postbus 500
2600 AM
Delft

Universities and technical universities

Rijksuniversiteit te Leiden
Acadameigebouw
PO Box 9500
2300 RA Leiden
Telephone: (71) 148333

Rijksuniversiteit te Groningen
PO Box 72
9700 AB Groningen
Telephone: (50) 119111

Rijksuniversiteit te Utrecht
PO Box 202
3512 HD Utrecht
Telephone: (30) 335722

Rijksuniversiteit te Rotterdam
PO Box 1738
3000 DR Rotterdam
Telephone: (10) 525511

Universiteit van Amsterdam (Gemeentelijke)
Postbus 19268
1000 GG Amsterdam
Telephone: (20) 5259111

Vrije Universiteit
PO Box 7161
1007 MC Amsterdam
Telephone: (20) 5489111

Rijksuniversiteit te Limburg
PO Box 616
6200 MD Maastricht
Telephone: (43) 888888

Katholieke Universiteit
Postbus 9102
6500 HC Nijmegen
Telephone: (80) 519333

Technische Hogeschool te Delft
Postbus 5
2600 AA Delft
Telephone: (15) 789111

Technische Hogeschool Twente
Postbus 217
7500 AE Enschede
Telephone: (53) 899111

Landbouwhogeschool
Postbus 9101
6700 HB Wageningen
Telephone: (8370) 89111

Technische Hogeschool te Eindhoven
Postbus 513
5600 MB Eindhoven
Telephone: (40) 479111

Insurance companies

Nationale Nederlanden
Pr. Beatrixlaan 15
2595 AK The Hague
Telephone: (70) 712712
Telex: 31585

Aegon N.V.
Churchillplein 1
2517 JW The Hague
Telephone: (70) 727272
Telex: 31657

Amev N.V.
Archimedeslaan 10
3584 BA Utrecht
Telephone: (30) 579111

Delta Lloyd Verzekeringen
Groep N.V.
Spaklerweg 4
1096 BA Amsterdam
Telephone: (20) 5949111
Telex: 18678

N.V. Assurantieconcern
Stad Rotterdam
Blaak 101
3011 GB Rotterdam
Telephone: (10) 141133
Telex: 23266

Centraal Beheer U.A.
Prins Willem Alexanderlaan 651
7312 GA Apeldoorn
Telephone: (55) 799111
Telex: 36366

Interpolis N.V.
Conservatoriumlaan 15
5037 DM Tilburg
Telephone: (13) 629111
Telex: 52291

Nieuw Rotterdam N.V.
Blaak 16
3011 TA Rotterdam
Telephone: (10) 143700
Telex: 21692

Royal Nederland
Verzekering Mij. N.V.
Coolsingel 139
3012 AG Rotterdam
Telephone: (10) 541911
Telex: 24029

VGCN/Zilveren Kruis U.A.
Biltstraat 196
3572 BR Utrecht
Telephone: (30) 715634

Zwitserleven
Apollolaan 153
1077 AS Amsterdam
Telephone: (20) 733232
Telex: 12570

UAP/Providentia N.V.
Keizersgracht 369–381
1016 EJ Amsterdam
Telephone: (20) 214545
Telex: 11245

Nederlandsche Credietverzekering Mij N.V.
(NCM)
Keizersgracht 271–277
1016 ED Amsterdam
Telephone: (20) 5539111
Telex: 11496

De Centrale N.V.
Rijnstraat 28
2515 XP Den Haag
Telephone: (70) 710710
Telex: 33142

Ohra, Onderlinge
Waarborgmij, U.A.
Groningensingel 51
6835 EC Arnhem
Telephone: (85) 249911
Telex: 75066

Zwolsche Algemeene N.V.
Oudenoord 3
3513 EG Utrecht
Telephone: (30) 330911
Telex: 47656

NOVO/VGNN
Nieuwe Veemarkt 10
8011 AH Zwolle
Telephone: (38) 210611
Telex: 42423

Goudse Verzekering Mij. N.V.
Stationsplein 3
2801 AK Gouda
Telephone: (1820) 41911
Telex: 20852

Zürich/VITA/Alpina
Oranjestraat 15
2514 JB Den Haag
Telephone: (70) 624401
Telex: 33273

Nutsziektekostenverzek
Loosduinseweg 9
2571 AA Den Haag
Telephone: (70) 100922

Stichting VGZ
St Annastraat 308
6525 HG Nijmegen
Telephone: (80) 566660

Main banks

De Nederlandsche Bank N.V.
Postbus 98
1000 AB Amsterdam
Telephone: (20) 5249111
Telex: 11355

Algemene Bank Nederland N.V.
Postbus 669
1000 EG Amsterdam
Telephone: (20) 299111
Telex: 11417

Amsterdam-Rotterdam Bank N.V.
Postbus 1220
1000 EH Amsterdam
Telephone: (20) 289393
Telex: 11006

Bank Mees & Hope N.V.
Postbus 293
1000 AG Amsterdam
Telephone: (20) 5279111
Telex: 11424

Banque Paribas Nederland N.V.
Postbus 274
1000 AG Amsterdam
Telephone: (20) 5204911
Telex: 11488

Credit Lyonnais Bank Nederland N.V.
Postbus 1045
3000 BA Rotterdam
Telephone: (10) 695911
Telex: 21366

F. van Lanschot Bankiers N.V.
Postbus 1021
5200 HC Den Bosch
Telephone: (73) 153911
Telex: 50641

Nederlandse Credietbank N.V.
Postbus 941
1000 AX Amsterdam
Telephone: (20) 556911
Telex: 14385

Nederlandsche Middenstandsbank N.V.
Postbus 1800
1000 BV Amsterdam
Telephone: (20) 5439111
Telex: 11402

Pierson, Heldring & Pierson NV
Postbus 243
1000 AE Amsterdam
Telephone: (20) 211188
Telex: 16388

Robobank Nederland
Postbus 17100
3500 HG Utrecht
Telephone: (30) 909111
Telex: 47700

Nederlandse Spaarbankbond
Postbus 3861
1081 AR Amsterdam
Telephone: (20) 221066
Telex: 126064

Medical bookshops

Academische Boek
Scheltema Holkema Vermeulen
Konigsplein 20–1017 BB
Amsterdam 1012 AH

Broese Kemink
Stadhuisberg 5
Postbus 38
Utrecht

Intermed
Witte de With Straat 5
3012 BK Rotterdam

New Zealand

There are good opportunities for private practice in New Zealand.

Government health organisations

Department of Health
PO Box 5013
Wellington

Department of Social Welfare
Private Bag
Wellington

Professional organisations

The New Zealand Medical Association
PO Box 156
Wellington 1

New Zealand Dental Association
369 Khyber Pass Road
Grafton
PO Box 28084
Auckland 5

The New Zealand Society of
Physiotherapists Inc.
National Office
PO Box 5198
Lambton Quay
Wellington

3rd Floor
Borthwick House
85 The Terrace
Wellington
Telephone: 735 768

New Zealand Society of Anaesthetists Inc.
Department of Anaesthesia
Waikato Hospital
Hamilton

Cardiac Society of New Zealand & Australia
Department of Cardiology
Greenlane Hospital
Auckland

Cancer Society of New Zealand
IBM House
The Terrace
Wellington

Emergency services and nursing

St John's Ambulance Service

Medical insurance

Southern Cross Medical Care Society
PO Box 9583
Auckland

Accident Compensation Corporation
Private Bag
Wellington

Medical insurance for practitioners

The Medical Protection Society Ltd
PO Box 156
Wellington

Medical Life Assurance Society
PO Box 1413
Wellington

Taxation offices

Inland Revenue Department
Private Bag
Wellington

Main banks

Royal Bank of New Zealand
ANZ Bank
CBA Bank
Westpac Bank

Medical bookshops

Medical Books (NZ) Ltd
PO Box 8565
Auckland

Medical Books (WGTN) Ltd
PO Box 7389
Wellington

Ackroyd's Medical and Nursing Books Ltd
PO Box 22–212
Christchurch

Peryer Educational Books Ltd
PO Box 6034
Christchurch

University Bookshop
19 High St
Auckland

University Bookshop
PO Box 6060
Dunedin

Bennetts Bookshop Ltd
PO Box 138
Palmerston North

Others

Whitcoulls Ltd
312 Lambton Quay
Wellington

The New Zealand Medical Journal
PO Box 5441
Dunedin

News and Views
PO Box 156
Wellington

Useful sources of information

Northern Locum Service
PO Box 34
166 Birkenhead
Auckland

Auckland Medical Bureau
469 Parnell Road
Auckland 1

Lower Hutt Locum Agency
PO Box 44
080 Lower Hutt

Palmerston North Locum Agency
PO Box 8056
Palmerston North

Sports organisations

New Zealand Council for
Recreation and Sport
PO Box 5122
Wellington

Fire and safety

Chubb (NZ) Ltd
98–100 Dixon Street
Wellington

New Zealand Fire Service
PO Box 2133
Wellington

New Zealand Safety Ltd
2 Regent Street
Petone
Wellington

Norway

The concentration of the population in one or two areas in Norway allows the existence of a few private practices and clinics outside the major towns. These are limited in number.

Professional organisations

Den Norske Laegforening
Inkognitogt 2
Oslo

Norske Fysiotherapeuters Forbund
Postboks 9590
Egertorget
Oslo 1

Medical insurance

Rikstrygdeverket
Drammensvn 60
Oslo 2

Taxation offices

Skattedirektoratet
Fredrik Selmersv 4
Oslo 6

Main banks

Den Norske Credeitbank
Oslo

Christiana Bank og Kredikasse
Oslo

Sparebanken Oslo Akershus
Oslo

Bergen Bank
Bergen

Medical bookshops

Tanum—Karl Johan A. S.
Karl Johans GT 43
0162 Oslo 1

Studia Universitetsbokhandel
Parkveien 1
Bergen

Useful sources of information

Telephone sales and directories

Teledirektoratet
Universitetsgt 2
Oslo 1

Sports organisations

Norges Idresttsforbund
Hauger Skolesv 1
1351 Rud

South Africa

There are many opportunities for private practice in South Africa. There is a comprehensive list of medical insurance schemes available from The Registrar of Medical Schemes in Pretoria.

Government health organisations

Department of Health and Welfare
Private Bag 19070
Captetown 8000

Department of Health and Welfare
Private Bag 63
Pretoria 0001 SA

Professional organisations

Medical Association of South Africa
PO Box 20272
Alkantrant
Pretoria 005

The Dental Association of South Africa
Private Bag 1
Houghton
Transvaal 2041

South African Association of Occupational
Therapists
PO Box 17289
Hillbrow
2038 Johannesburg

South African Society of Physiotherapy
PO Box 47238
Parklands
2121 Johannesburg

South African Association of Registered
Podiatrists
42 Rustenburg
126 Currie Road
Durban 4001

South African Speech and Hearing
Association
PO Box 31782
Braamfountein 2017

Taxation offices

Receiver of Revenue
PO Box 1051
Johannesburg 2000

Private independent hospitals and clinics

The Representative Association of
Private Hospitals
c/o Box 45175
Mayfair 2108

Screening and diagnostic

South African Institute for
Medical Research
Hospital Hill
Johannesburg 2000

Medical bookshops

Westdene Services
PO Box 7710
Johannesburg 2000

Clinician C.A.S.A. Journal
Editor
PO Box 706
Bethlehem 9700

Useful sources of information

Community care

The Stroke Aid Association
PO Box 51283
Raedene 2124
Johannesburg

South African Council for the Deaf
Lonsbank Building
Bree Street
Johannesburg 2001

The South African Association of Inherited
Disorders
c/o Johannesburg Hospital
Parktown
Johannesburg

Fire and safety

South African Bureau of Standards
PO Box 61092
Marshaltown 2107
Johannesburg

Health premises building consultants
Leasedoc
Durdoc Centre
Smith Street
Durban 4000

Sweden

There are limited opportunities for private practice as medical care is generally financed by the Government.

Government organisations

Ministry of Health and Social Affairs
S-10333 Stockholm

Professional organisations

Sveriges Lakarforbund—The Swedish Medical Association
Box 5610
Villagatan 5
11486 Stockholm
Telephone: 46 822 4740

The Swedish Dental Association
Box 5843
102 48 Stockholm

Forbundet Sveriges Arbetsterapeuter—Occupational Therapists
Box 36
13106 Nacka
Ryssviksvagen 2
Telephone: 08/716 28 50

Legitimerade Sjukgymnasters—Physical Therapy Association
Riksforbund
Box 3196
Wallingatan 5
10363 Stockholm

Main banks

Skandinaviska Enskilda Banken
Kungstradgardsgatan 8
Stockholm S-111 47

Medical bookshop

Almqvist and Wikselle
Gamla Brogatan 26
Stockholm

Useful sources of information

Svenska Roda Korset
Box 27316
S-102 54 Stockholm

Radda Barnen
Box 27320
S-102 54 Stockholm

The Swedish Institute for the Handicapped
Box 303
16126 Bromma
Telephone: 08 87 91 40

Telephone sales and directories

Televerket
S-123 86 Farsta

Postverket
Vasagatan 28–34
S-105 00 Stockholm

Private recruitment agency

Praktikertjanst AB
PO Box 1304
S-11183 Stockholm

Switzerland

Switzerland has no centralised Ministry of Health. All practical matters are dealt with by the individual cantons. Medicine is practised privately throughout Switzerland.

Government health organisations

Office federal de la sante publique
Postfach 2644/Bollwerk 27
CH-3001 Bern

Professional organisations: medical organisations

Schweizerische Aerzteorganisation
(Institutions du corps médical suisse)

Generalsekretariat
(Secrétariat général)

Elfenstrasse 18
3000 Bern 16
Switzerland
Telephone: 031/43. 55. 43

Société médicale de la Suisse romande
1 route d'Oron
1010 Lausanne
Telephone: 021/32. 16. 74

Ordine dei medici del cantone del Ticino
Via Besso 41
6900 Lugano
Telephone: 091/56. 45. 73

Schweiz. Krankenhausinstitut (SKI)
(Institut suisse des hôpitaux (ISH)
(Swiss hospital organization)
Pfrundweg 14
5001 Aarau
Telephone: 064/24. 71. 61

Medical insurance

Union des Federations suisses de caisse maladie
Romerstrasse 20
CH-4500 Solothurn

Taxation offices

Federal Tax Administration
Eigerstrasse 65
CH-3003 Berne

Main banks

Bank Julius Baer & Co., Ltd.
Sarasin (UK) Ltd.
Swiss Volksbank
Credit Suisse
Swiss Bank Corporation
Union Bank of Switzerland

Medical bookshop

Librairie Payot
1 Rue de Bourg
Ch-1002 Lausanne

United Kingdom

There are many useful organisations and sources of reference for the health care professions. It is advisable to contact the professional organisation first before starting private practice in order to establish their guidelines and also to contract the local council offices of the region.

Government organisations

Department of Health and Social Security
Alexander Fleming House
Elephant and Castle
London SE1 6BY
Telephone: 01-407 5522

Department of Trade and Industry
Floor 11
Millbank Tower
London SW1 4QU
Telephone: 01-211 6088

Council for the Professions Supplementary to Medicine
Park House
184 Kennington Park Road
London SE11 4BU
Telephone: 01-582 0866

Health Education Council
78 New Oxford Street
London WC1A 1AH
Telephone: 01-637 1881

Health Services Commissioner for England (Ombudsman)
Church House
Great Smith Street
London SW1
Telephone: 01-212 7676

Health Services Commissioner for Wales
3rd Floor
Queen's Court
Plymouth Street
Cardiff CF1 4DA
Telephone: 0222 394621

Manpower Services Commission
19–29 Woburn Place
London WC1
Telephone: 01-837 1288

Medical Practices Committee
Tavistock House South
London WC1
Telephone: 01-388 6471

National Consumer Council
18 Queen Anne's Gate
London SW1 9AA
Telephone: 01-222 9501

Small Firms Division of the Department of Trade & Industry
Ashdown House
127 Victoria Street
London SW1E 6RB
Telephone: 01-212 8667

Organisations representing patients

Association of Community Health Councils for England and Wales
362 Euston Road
London NW1
Telephone: 01-388 4814

Association of Welsh Community Health Councils
5 Chalybeate Street
Aberystwyth
Dyfed
Wales
Telephone: 9070 4760

Professional organisations

The British Chiropractic Association
5 First Avenue
Chelmsford
Essex CM1 1RX
Telephone: 0245 358487

The British Medical Association
BMA House
Tavistock Square
London WC1
Telephone: 01-387 4499

The British Orthopaedic Association
35 Lincoln's Inn Fields
Telephone: 01-405 6507

The British Red Cross Society
9 Grosvenor Crescent
London SW1
Telephone: 01-235 5454

The British Society of Osteopathy
1 Suffolk Street
London SW1Y 4HG
Telephone: 01-930 9254

The British Association of Occupational
Therapists
20 Rede Place
London W2 4TU
Telephone: 01-229 9738

The Chartered Society of Physiotherapy
14 Bedford Row
London WC1
Telephone: 01-242 1941

The College of Speech Therapists
6 Lechmere Road
London NW2
Telephone: 01-459 8521

The Council for Postgraduate Medical
Education
7 Marylebone Road
London NW1
Telephone: 01-323 1299

The General Medical Council
44 Hallam Street
Portland Place
London W1N 6AE

The Organisation of Chartered
Physiotherapists in Private Practice
11 The Larches
Benfleet
Essex SS7 4NR
Telephone: 0702 715549

The Royal College of General Practitioners
14 Prince's Gate
London SW7
Telephone: 01-584 6262

The Royal College of Nursing
Henrietta Place
London W1
Telephone: 01-580 2646

The Royal College of Obstetricians &
Gynaecologists
27 Sussex Place
London NW1
Telephone: 01-580 2646

The Royal College of Physicians
11 St Andrew's Place
London NW1
Telephone: 01-935 1174

The Royal College of Surgeons
35 Lincoln's Inn Fields
London WC2
Telephone: 01-405 3474

The Society of Chiropodists
53 Welbeck Street
London W1
Telephone: 01-486 3381

The Society of Radiographers
14 Upper Wimpole Street
London W1
Telephone: 01-935 2626

Alternative medicine organisations

The British Homeopathic Association
27A Devonshire Street
London W1N 1RJ
Telephone: 01-935 2163

The British Society of Medical and Dental
Hypnosis
PO Box 6
Ashtead
Surrey KT21 2HJ

The National Federation of Spiritual Healers
Old Manor Farm Studio
Church Street
Sunbury-on-Thames
Middlesex TW16 6RG
Telephone: Sunbury 83164

*Organisations representing medical
practitioners*

British Medical Association
BMA House
Tavistock Square
London WC1
Telephone: 01-387 4499

British Medical Association
BMA Welsh Office
195 Newport Road
Cardiff CF2 1UE
Telephone: 0222 485 336

Dentists Provident Society
63 Wimpole Street
London W1
Telephone: 01-487 4814

Hospital Consultants & Specialists
Association
The Old Court House
London Road
Ascot
Berkshire SL5 7EN
Telephone: Ascot 25052

Medical Practitioners Union
10–26A Jamestown Road
London NW1 7DT
Telephone: 01-267 4422

Medical Defence Union
3 Devonshire Place
London W1N 2EA
Telephone: 01-486 6181

Medical Practices Committee
Tavistock House South
London WC1
Telephone: 01-388 6471

Medical Protection Society
50 Hallam Street
London W1N 6DE
Telephone: 01-637 0541

Medical insurance

Allied Medical Assurance Services Ltd
Brettenham House
Lancaster Place
London WC2
Telephone: 01-379 6161

British United Provident Association
(BUPA)
Provident House
Essex Street
London WC2R 3BR
Telephone: 01-836 1048
               01-353 5212

BUPA branch offices
Northern Bank House
10 High Street
Belfast BTA 2BJ
Telephone: Belfast (0232) 24224

Belmont House
40 Vicarage Road
Edgbaston
Birmingham B15 3DZ
Telephone: 021-455 8821

Heron House
8–10 Christchurch Road
Bournemouth BH1 3NP
Telephone: Bournemouth (0202) 294741

Gresham House
44 North Road
Brighton BN1 1YT
Telephone: Brighton (0273) 608121

Inter City House
Victoria Street
Bristol BS1 6BH
Telephone: Bristol (0272) 214511

Provident House
122 High Street
Bromley BR1 1TB
Telephone: 01-466 6531

Kett House
Station Road
Cambridge CB1 2JP
Telephone: Cambridge (0223) 64441

Alliance House
High Street
Cardiff CF1 2RR
Telephone: Cardiff (0222) 25442

132 Station Road
Chingford
London E4 6AE
Telephone: 01-524 5281

BUPA House
116 Dundas Street
Edinburgh EH3 5EC
Telephone: 031 557 3400

Devon House
3 Paris Street
Exeter EX1 2JE
Telephone: Exeter (0392) 77234

Charlotte House
78 Queen Street
Glasgow G1 3DL
Telephone: 041-248 7554

Raebarn House
Northolt Road
South Harrow HA2 0DT
Telephone: 01-864 5511

Vicar Lane House
5 Templar Street
Leeds LS2 7NZ
Telephone: Leeds (0532) 444041

Concourse House
Lime Street
Liverpool L69 1PN
Telephone: 051-709 6946

St Andrew's House
Portland Street
Manchester M1 3LU
Telephone: 061-236 7335

Crown House
London Road
Morden
Surrey SM4 5EH
Telephone: 01-542 2231

Commercial Union House
29–47 Pilgrim Street
Newcastle NE1 6QE
Telephone: Newcastle (0632) 29751

Clerical, Medical Assurance House
25 St James's Street
Nottingham NG1 5AY
Telephone: Nottingham (0602) 49891

Prama House
267 Banbury Road
Oxford OX2 7JB
Telephone: Oxford (0865) 52002

Provident House
Bridge Street
Staines
Middlesex TW18 4TL
Telephone: Staines (0784) 59361

Crusader Insurance PLC
13 Tower Place
London EC3
Telephone: 01-621 0684

Crusader Insurance PLC
103 Jermyn Street
London SW1
Telephone: 01-930 0952

Crusader Insurance PLC
Reigate
Surrey RH2 8BL
Telephone: 073 72 42424

L.A.M.P.S. Insurance
45 Queen's Square
Corby
Northants NN17 1PD
Telephone: 0536 201661

Milas Ltd
45 Queen's Square
Corby
Northants NN17 1PD
Telephone: 0536 201661

Private Patients Plan
Eynsham House
Tunbridge Wells
Kent
Telephone: 0892 40111

Private Patients Plan
Tavistock House South
Tavistock Square
London WC1
Telephone: 01-387 5166
         01-388 2468

Western Provident Association Ltd (WPA)
Culverhouse
Culver Street
Bristol BS1 5JE
Telephone: 0272 273241

WPA branch offices
26 Park Street
Bristol BS1 5JB
Telephone: 0272 273241

13 North Park Road
Harrogate
North Yorks HG1 5PD
Telephone: 0423 62276

4 Salisbury Road
Leicester LE1 7QR
Telephone: 0533 551318

160 Piccadilly
London W1V 0BX
Telephone: 01-409 0414

29 Castle Street
Reading
Berkshire RG1 7SL
Telephone: 0734 54141

Taxation offices

HM Inspectors of Taxes
Inland Revenue
4 Grosvenor Place
London SW1
Telephone: 01-235 9991

Main banks

Lloyds Bank PLC
National Westminster Bank PLC
Midland Bank
Barclays Bank PLC
Royal Bank of Scotland

Other sources of finance

Prudential Assurance Co. Ltd
Welsh Development Agency
West Midland Enterprise Board
Charterhouse Group
Manpower Services

Private independent hospitals and clinics

Alexandra Hospital
Mill Lane
Cheadle
Cheshire SK8 2PX
Telephone: 061-428 3656

All Hallows Hospital
Ditchingham
Bungay
Suffolk NR35 2QL
Telephone: Bungay 2728

AMI American Medical International
Health Care Ltd
4 Cornwall Terrace
Regents Park
London NW1 4AP
Telephone: 01-486 1266

Battersea Mission Varicose Clinic
14 York Road
London SW11
Telephone: 01-228 6663

Beechwood Private Clinic
Norton Church Road
Sheffield S8 8JQ
Telephone: 0742 74811

Benenden Chest Hospital
Benenden
Cranbrook
Kent TN17 4AX
Telephone: Cranbrook 240333

The Blackheath Hospital
40–42 Lee Terrace
London SE3 QUD
Telephone: 01-318 7722

Bowden House Clinic
London Road
Harrow-on-the-Hill
Middlesex
Telephone: 01-864 0221

British Home & Hospital for Incurables
Crown Lane
Streatham
London SW16 3JB
Telephone: 01-670 8261

BUPA Hospital
Bushey
Heathbourne Road
Bushey
Watford WD2 1RD
Telephone: 01-950 9090

BUPA Hospital Cardiff
Croescadam Road
Pentwyn
Cardiff CF2 7ZL
Telephone: 0222 735515

BUPA Hospital Manchester
Russell Road
Whalley Range
Manchester M16 8AJ
Telephone: 061-226 0112

BUPA Hospital Harpenden
Ambrose Lane
Harpenden AL5 4BP
Telephone: 05827 63191

BUPA Murrayfield Hospital
Holmwood Drive
Thingwall
Wirral
Merseyside
Telephone: 051-648 7000

BUPA Hospital Norwich
Old Watton Road
Colney
Norwich NR4 7TD
Telephone: 0603 56181

BUPA Hospital Portsmouth
Bartons Road
Havant
Hants PO9 5NP
Telephone: 0705 454511

C.G. Jung Clinic of the Society of Analytical
Psychology Ltd
1 Daleham Gardens
London NW3
Telephone: 01-435 7696

Catisfield House Convalescent Home for
Women
55 The Drive
Hove
E. Sussex BN3 3PF
Telephone: Brighton 736036

Charter Clinic
1–5 Radnor Walk
London SW3 4PB
Telephone: 01-351 1272

Chaucer Hospital
Nackington Road
Canterbury
Kent CT4 7AR
Telephone: 0227 455466

Cheadle Royal Hospital
Cheadle
Cheshire SK8 3DG
Telephone: 061-428 9511

Chiltern Hospital
Great Missenden
Bucks HP16 0EN
Telephone: 024 06 6565

Churchill Clinic
80 Lambeth Road
London SE1 7PU
Telephone: 01-928 5633

Claremont Nursing Home
401 Sandygate Road
Sheffield S10 5UB
Telephone: 0742 302953

Clementine Churchill Hospital
Sudbury Hill
Harrow
Middlesex HA1 3RX
Telephone: 01-422 3464

Clevedon Convalescent Homes
Belmont Convalescent Home
Chapel Hill
Clevedon
Avon BS21 7LL
Telephone: 0272 872031

Clinic of Psychotherapy
26 Belsize Square
London NW3
Telephone: 01-903 6455

Community Hospitals PLC
The Merton Centre
45 St Peter's Street
Bedford MK40 2UB
Telephone: 0234 67555

College of St Barnabas
Blackberry Lane
Lingfield
Surrey
Telephone: Dormans Park 260

Convent Hospital
748 Mansfield Road
Woodthorpe
Nottingham NG5 3FZ
Telephone: Nottingham 268244

Cromwell Hospital
Cromwell Road
London SW5 0TU
Telephone: 01-370 4233

David Lewis Centre for Epilepsy
Nr Alderley Edge
Cheshire SK9 7UD
Telephone: Mobberley 2613

Devonshire Hospital
Devonshire Street
London W1N 1RF
Telephone: 01-486 7131

Dispensaire Francais
6 Osnaburgh Street
London NW1 3DH
Telephone: 01-387 5132

Dunedin Hospital
16 Bath Road
Reading RG1 6NB
Telephone: 0734 587676

Emergency Bed Service
Fielden House
28 London Bridge Street
London SE1 9SG
Telephone: 01-407 7181

Enham Village Centre
The White House
Enham-Alamein
Andover
Hants
Telephone: Andover 51551

Evelyn Hospital
4 Trumpington Road
Cambridge CB2 2AF
Telephone: 0223 353401

Fitzwilliam Hospital
Milton Way
South Bretton
Peterborough PE3 8YQ
Telephone: 0733 261717

Galsworthy House
Kingston Hill
Kingston-upon-Thames
Surrey KT2 7LX
Telephone: 01-549 9861

Gatwick Park Hospital
Porey Cross Road
Horley
Surrey RH6 0BB
Telephone: 0293 785511

Harley Street Clinic
35 Weymouth Street
London W1N 4BJ
Telephone: 01-935 7700

Hayes Grove Priory Hospital
Prestons Road
Hayes
Bromley
Kent BR2 7AS
Telephone: 01-462 7722

HCA
49 Wigmore Street
London W1H 9LE
Telephone: 01-937 7185

Holy Cross Hospital
Haslemere
Surrey GU27 1NG
Telephone: 0428 3311

Hospital of St John of God
Scorton
Richmond
N. Yorks DL10 6EB
Telephone: Richmond 811536

Hospital of St John & St Elizabeth
60 Grove End Road
St John's Wood
London NW8 9NH
Telephone: 01-286 5126

Hospital Saturday Fund
192–198 Vauxhall Bridge Road
Victoria
London SW1V 1EE
Telephone: 01-828 0836

Invalid Children's Aid Association
126 Buckingham Palace Road
London SW1
Telephone: 01-730 9891

Italian Hospital
Queen Street
London WC1N 3AN
Telephone: 01-831 6961

Jewish Home & Hospital at Tottenham
295 High Road
London N15 4RT
Telephone: 01-800-5138

King Edward VII Hospital
Beaumont House
Beaumont Street
London W1N 2AA
Telephone: 01-486-4411

King Edward VII Hospital
Midhurst
W. Sussex
Telephone: 073 081 2341

Lansdowne Private Hospital
67 Lansdowne Road
Bournemouth BH1 1RW
Telephone: 0202 291866

Leicester & County Convalescent Homes
Society
84 Northampton Street
Leicester
Telephone: 0533 20617

Lingfield Hospital School
Lingfield
Surrey
Telephone: 0342 832243

London Clinic
20 Devonshire Place
London W1N 2DH
Telephone: 01-935 4444

London Clinic of Psycho-Analysis
63 New Cavendish Street
London W1
Telephone: 01-580 4952

Maghull Homes
Maghull
Merseyside L31 8BR
Telephone: 051-526 4133

Manchester & Salford Hospital Saturday
Fund
43–45 Lever Street
Manchester M60 7HP
Telephone: 061–236 1901

Manor House Hospital
North End Road
Golders Green
London NW11
Telephone: 01-455 6601

Metropolitan Hospital Saturday Fund
40 High Street
Teddington
Middlesex TW11 8EW
Telephone: 01-977 4154

Murrayfield Hospital
122 Corstorphine Road
Edinburgh
Telephone: 031-334 0363

National Society for Epilepsy
Chalfont Centre for Epilepsy
Chalfont St Peter
Bucks
Telephone: Chalfont St Giles 3991

New Victoria Hospital
184 Coombe Lane West
Kingston-upon-Thames
Surrey
Telephone: 01-949 1661

Nestor Medical Services
56 Kingsway
London WC28 6DX
Telephone: 01-404 3122

Fairfield House (Head Office)
Chesham Road
Tring
Herts
Telephone: 024-029 797

North Wales Medical Centre
Queen's Road
Craig-y-Don
Llandudno
Gwynedd LL30 1UD
Telephone: Llandudno 79031

Nottingham General Dispensary
12 Broad Street
Nottingham
Telephone: 0602 473333

Nuffield Hospitals
Aldwych House
71–91 Aldwych
London WC18 4EE
Telephone: 01-404 0601

Paddocks Private Hospital
Aylesbury Road
Princes Risborough
Bucks
Telephone: 084 44 6951-9

Park Hospital
Sherwood Lodge Drive
Alton
Nottingham
Telephone: 0602 20811

Portland Hospital for Women and Children
Great Portland Street
London W1N 5HA
Telephone: 01-580 4400

Post Office & Civil Service Sanatorium
Society
63 Catherine Place
London SW1E 6HE
Telephone: 01-834 5022

Princess Grace Hospital
45–52 Nottingham Place
London W1M 5FD
Telephone: 01-486 1234

Princess Louise Scottish Hospital
Erskine
Bishopton
Renfrewshire PA7 5PU
Telephone: 041-812 1100

Princess Margaret Hospital
Osborne Road
Windsor
Berks SL4 5EJ
Telephone: 0753 68292

Priory Hospital
Priory Lane
Roehampton
London SW15 5JJ
Telephone: 01-876 8261

Priory Hospital
Priory Road
Edgbaston
Birmingham B5 7UG
Telephone: 021-440 2323

Queen Alexandra Hospital Home
Gifford House
Boundary Road
Worthing
W. Sussex
Telephone: 0903 202486

Queen Victoria Memorial Home of Rest
Wheeldon Avenue
Derby
Telephone: 0332 45248

Railway Convalescent Homes
6/8 Hampshire Terrace
Portsmouth PO1 2UD
Telephone: 0705 736961

The Retreat
York YO1 5BN
Telephone: 0904 412551

Ross Hall Hospital
221 Crookston Road
Glasgow G51 3NQ
Telephone: 041-882 9092

Royal Hospital & Home for Incurables
Putney
West Hill
London SW15 3SW
Telephone: 01-788 4511

Royal Masonic Hospital
Ravenscourt Park
London W6 0TN
Telephone: 01-748 4611

Royal Star & Garter Home for Disabled
Sailors, Soldiers and Airmen
Richmond-upon-Thames, Surrey
Telephone: 01-940 3314

St Andrew's Hospital
Northampton
Telephone: 0604 29696

St Anthony's Hospital
London Road
North Cheam
Surrey
Telephone: 01-330 3351

St David's Home for Disabled
Ex-Servicemen
Castlebar Hill
Ealing
London W5
Telephone: 01-997 5121

St Joseph's Hospital
Burlington Lane
Chiswick
London W4 2QE
Telephone: 01-994 4641

St Luke's Hospital for the Clergy
14 Fitzroy Square
London W1P 6AH
Telephone: 01-388 4954

St Margaret's Home for Invalids
Myreslawgreen
Hawick
Roxburghshire
Telephone: 0450 3162

St Mary's Hospital
Lanark
Telephone: 0555 2393

St Mary's Nursing Home for Elderly
Women
Stone
Staffs
Telephone: 813 894

St Michael's Hospital
Hayle
Cornwall
Telephone: 753234

St Saviour's Hospital
73 Seabrook Road
Hythe
Kent CT21 5QW
Telephone: 0303 65581

St Teresa's Hospital
12 The Downs
Wimbledon
London SW20 8HS
Telephone: 01-947 3142

St Vincent's Orthopaedic Hospital
Eastcote
Pinner
Middlesex
Telephone: 01-866 0151

Sloane Hospital
125–133 Albemarle Road
Beckenham
Kent BR3 2HS
Telephone: 01-466 6911

Ticehurst House Private Clinic
Ticehurst
Wadhurst
E. Sussex
Telephone: Ticehurst 200391

Trinity Hospice
30 Clapham Common
North Side
London SW4 0RN
Telephone: 01-622 9481

The Turner Home
Dingle Head
Liverpool 8
Telephone: 051-727 4177

Unstead Park
Unstead Heath
Godalming
Surrey
Telephone: 0483 892061

Warwickshire Orthopaedic Hospital
The Chase
Old Milverton Lane
Leamington Spa
Warwickshire CV32 6RW
Telephone: 27971

Wellington Hospital
Wellington Place
London NW8 9LE
Telephone: 01-586 5959

West Kirby Residential School
West Kirby
Wirral
Merseyside
Telephone: 051-632 3201

West Sussex Clinic
48 Shelley Road
Worthing
W. Sussex BN11 4DB
Telephone: 0903 213711

Winchester Private Clinic
The Nursing Home
Bereweeke Road
Winchester, Hants
Telephone: Hants 54774

Working Men's Club & Institute Union
Club Union House
251–256 Upper Street
London N1 1RY
Telephone: 01-226 0221

Yorkshire Clinic
Bradford Road
Bingley
W. Yorks BD16 1TW
Telephone: Bradford 560311

Medical personnel agencies and bureau services

British Nursing Association
443/470 Oxford Street
London W1R
Telephone: 01-629 9030

British United Provident Association
(BUPA)
BUPA Nursing Services
36 Dover Street
London W1X 3EB
Telephone: 01-629 4233

BUPA Nursing Services
Harrow
Middlesex
Telephone: 01-423 6272

BUPA Nursing Services
Bromley
Kent
Telephone: 01-460 5858

BUPA nursing

Birmingham
1st Floor
Unicorn House
Smallbrook Queensway
Birmingham B5 4HE
Telephone: 021-632 6476/7

Bristol
6th Floor
Inter City House
Victoria Street
Bristol BS1 6BH
Telephone: (0272) 277170

Cardiff
BUPA Hospital Cardiff
Croescadarn Road
Pentwyn
Cardiff CF2 7XL
Telephone: (0222) 735705

Leeds
2nd Floor
Vicar Lane House
5 Templar Street
Leeds LS2 7NZ
Telephone: (0532) 450611
or (0274) 394449 (Bradford)

Liverpool
21 Rodney Street
Liverpool L1 9EF
Telephone: 051-709 0011

London
33 Heddon Street
London W1R 7LL
Telephone: 01-734 8978
or 01-423 6272 (Harrow)
and 01-460 5858 (Bromley)

Manchester
9 St John Street
Manchester M3 4DW
Telephone: 061-834 1155

Norwich
BUPA Hospital Norwich
The Old Dairy
Old Watton Road
Colney
Norwich NR4 7TD
Telephone: (0603) 505751 and 505754

Nottingham
92 Friar Lane
Nottingham NG1 6EB
Telephone: (0602) 415315

Oxford
Felstead House
23 Banbury Road
Oxford OX2 6PD
Telephone: (0865) 56624

BUPA medical centres

London
Webb House
210 Pentonville Road
Kings Cross
London N1 9TA
Telephone: General enquiries
01-278 4651/01-837 6484
Telex: 268508
Men's Unit appointments 01-837 7055

London
Battle Bridge House
300 Grays Inn Road
London WC1X 8DU
Telephone: 01-278 4651/01-837 6484
Women's Unit appointments 01-837 7055

Birmingham
Unicorn House
29 Smallbrook Queensway
Birmingham B5 4HE
Telephone: 021-632 6738

Brentwood
Hartswood Hospital
Warley Road
Brentwood
Essex CM13 3HR
Telephone: (0277) 232525

Bristol
Stafford Lodge
The Chesterfield Hospital
Clifton Hill
Bristol BS8 1BP
Telephone: (0272) 731433

Bushey
BUPA Hospital Bushey
Heathbourne Road
Bushey
Watford WD2 1RD
Telephone: 01-950 9090

Cardiff
BUPA Hospital Cardiff
Croescadarn Road
Pentwyn
Cardiff CF2 7XL
Telephone: (0222) 735515

Glasgow
Axton House
295 Fenwick Road
Giffnock
Glasgow G46 6UH
Telephone: 041-638 4445

Leeds
81 Clarendon Road
Leeds LS2 9PJ
Telephone: (0532) 436735

Manchester
9 St John Street
Manchester M3 4DW
Telephone: 061-833 9362

Norwich
BUPA Hospital Norwich
Old Watton Road
Colney
Norwich NR4 7TD
Telephone: (0603) 56181

Nottingham
Clawson Lodge
403 Mansfield Road
Nottingham NG5 2DP
Telephone: (0602) 622826

Sutton Coldfield
Little Aston Hospital
Little Aston
Sutton Coldfield
West Midlands B74 3UP
Telephone: 021-353 2444

Personnel and Bureau Agencies

Commumlink
Private Speech Therapy
Referral Service
2 Paul Court
Fairfield Road
London N18 2PJ
Telephone: 01-884 1210

Corinth Medical Services
96 High Street
Bushey
Herts
Telephone: 01-950 6105

Era Agency
14 Great Portland Street
London W1
Telephone: 01-580 8915

Nightingale Medical Personnel Services
7 Aragon Avenue
Thames Ditton
Surrey
Telephone: 01-398 4462

United Medical Enterprises Ltd
18 Grosvenor Gardens
London SW1
Telephone: 01-730 4511

X-ray and screening services

Cardiac Recorders Ltd
34 Scarborough Road
London N4 4LU
Telephone: 01-272 9212

Cavendish X-Rays Ltd
6 Dorset Street
London W1
Telephone: 01-935 3617

Charter Clinic
1/7 Radnor Walk
London SW3
Telephone: 01-353 1272

Churchill Clinic
80 Lambeth Road
London SE1 7PU
Telephone: 01-928 5633

Ladbroke Clinic
6 Ladbroke Road
London W11
Telephone: 01-229 3832
            01-727 2080

Mobile Radiography Services Ltd
3 Grosvenor Road
Brentford
Telephone: 01-568 2145

Portable X-rays Ltd
3 Spanish Place
London W1
Telephone: 01-637 8938

PPP Medical Centre
99 New Cavendish Street
London W1M 7FQ
Telephone: 01-637 8941

Worldwide X-ray
23 Bryanston Square
London W1
Telephone: 01-724 3095

Health clinics and hydros

Champneys at Tring Ltd
Tring
Herts
Telephone: 044 27 3351

Champneys at Stobo
Stobo Castle Peebleshire
Scotland
Telephone: 0721 6249

Enton Hall
Enton
Godalming
Surrey
Telephone: 042 879 2233

Forest Mere
Liphook
Hampshire
Telephone: 0428 722051

Grayshott Hall
Headley Road
Grayshott
Hindhead
Surrey
Telephone: 042 873 4331

Henlow Grange
Henlow
Bedfordshire
Telephone: 0462 811111

Inglewood Health Hydro Ltd
Kintbury
Newbury
Berks
Telephone: 0488 2022

Ragdale Hall
Ragdale
Melton Mowbray
Leics
Telephone: 066 475 831/411

Shrubland Hall
Coddenham
Ipswich
Suffolk
Telephone: 0473 830404

Tyringham
Newport Pagnell
Bucks
Telephone: 0908 610430

Medical bookshops

James F. Bisset
Aberdeen Royal Infirmary
Forresterhill
Aberdeen

Robinson's Bookshop
11 Bond Street
Brighton

Georges
89 Park Street
Bristol

John Wright
44 Triangle West
Bristol

Heffers
Trinity Street
Cambridge

Lears
13–17 Royal Arcade
Cardiff

University Bookshop
Student's Union Building
Senghennydd Road
Cardiff

University Bookshop
95 Nethergate
Dundee

Donald Ferrier Limited
5–18 Teviot Place
Edinburgh

James Thin Booksellers
South Bridge
Edinburgh

John Smith and Son
57–61 St Vincent Street
Glasgow

John Smith and Son
John McIntyre Building
University of Glasgow
Glasgow

Austicks Medical Bookshop
57 Great George Street
Leeds

University Bookshop
University Road
Leicester

Parrys Books
Brownlow Hill
Liverpool

Dillons University Bookshop
1 Malet Street
London WC1

W. and G. Foyle
113–119 Charing Cross Road
London WC2

Kimptons Medical Bookshop
205 Great Portland Street
London W1

H. K. Lewis
136 Gower Street
London WC1

Modern Book Company
15–21 Praed Street
London W2

Haigh and Hochland
Oxford Road
Manchester

Thornes University Bookshop
63 and 67 Percy Street
Newcastle

University Bookshop (Nottingham)
Queen's Medical Centre
Clifton Boulevard
University Hospital
Nottingham

B. H. Blackwell Ltd
48 Broad Street
Oxford

W. Hartley Seed
152–160 West Street
Sheffield

Bowes and Bowes
The University
Highfield
Southampton

Useful sources of information

Ambulance services

Acme Private Ambulance Service
144 Old Brompton Road
London SW7
Telephone: 01-373 1820

Ambuline Private Ambulance Service
23 Redwood Close
Kings Norton
Birmingham
Telephone: 021-459 2342

Ambu-Save Ambulance Service
5/15 Collingham Place
London SW5
Telephone: 01-373 6801

A–Z Winston Ambulance Services
Heath House
Bexley Heath
Kent
Telephone: 01-303 6288

AID Ambulance International & Domestic
Ltd
Group House
Moss Lane
Rochdale
Lancs
Telephone: (0706) 53137

British Euro Medi-Vac Services
Telephone: 01-318 7307

Greater Manchester & Pennine Private
Ambulance
Paragon House
Smithy Bridge
Littleborough
Telephone: Littleborough 78317

Inter-County Ambulance Service
The Ambulance Station
Gravel Hill
Chalfont St Peter
Bucks
Telephone: (0753) 883432

Mexedel Ltd
Operation Centre
Capital House
2–4 Heigham Street
Norwich
Telephone: (0603) 630066

Meditrans Ambulance Ltd
Hospital of St John & Elizabeth
Grove End Road
London NW8
Telephone: 01-289 6180

St John's Ambulance
1 Grosvenor Crescent
London SW1
Telephone: 01-235 5231

Sovereign Services
Head Office
Gatwick Airport
Telephone: Crawley 547932

Back associations

The Osteopathic Association of Great
Britain
3 The Drive
Kettering
Northants

The Back Pain Association
Grundy House
31–33 Park Road
Teddington TW11 0AB
Telephone: 01-977 5474/5

The British Association of Manipulative
Medicine
22 Wimpole Street
London W1 7AD
Telephone: 01-637 0491

The British Chiropractors Association
5 First Avenue
Chelmsford
Essex CM1 1EX
Telephone: 0245 358487

The Chartered Society of Physiotherapy
14 Bedford Row
London WC1
Telephone: 01-242 1941

The Manipulation Association of Manual
Medicine
14 Bedford Row
London WC1
Telephone: 01-242 1941

The International Federation of Manual
Medicine
28 Wimpole Street
London W1 7AD

Children's organisations

Cystic Fibrosis Research Trust
Alexandra House
5 Blythe Road
Bromley
Kent BR1 2RS
Telephone: 01-464 7211

Down's Syndrome Children's Association
4 Oxford Street
London W1R 1PA
Telephone: 01-580 0511

National Association for the Welfare of
Children in Hospital
7 Exton Street
London SE1 8UE
Telephone: 01-261 1738

National Childbirth Trust
9 Queensborough Terrace
London W2 3TB
Telephone: 01-221 3833

Pre-School Playgroups Association
Alford House
Aveline Street
London SE11 5DH
Telephone: 01-582 8871

Disabled—amenities and information

Banstead Place Mobility Centre
Park Road
Banstead
Surrey
Telephone: 073 73 51674

Bristol Aids Centre
172–174 Kellaway Avenue
Horfield
Bristol B56 7YQ

British Amputee Sports Association
2 Bell Road
Cosham
Portsmouth POX 3NX

British Ski Club for the Disabled
Corton House
Corton
Warminster
Wiltshire BA12 0SZ
Telephone: 0985 50321

Central Council for the Disabled
25 Mortimer Street
London W1
Telephone: 01-637 5400

DIAL
National Association of Disablement
Information and Advice Services
117 High Street
Clay Cross
Chesterfield
Telephone: 0246 864498

Disabled Drivers Association
Ashwellthorpe
Norwich NR16 1RX
Telephone: 050841 449

John Grooms Association for the Disabled—
Holidays for the Disabled
10 Gloucester Drive
Finsbury Park
London N4 2LP
Telephone: 01-802 7272

Information Service for Disabled People
Northern Ireland
2 Annadale Avenue
Belfast BT7 3JH
Telephone: 0232 640011

Mary Marlborough Lodge for the Disabled
Nuffield Orthopaedic Centre
Headington
Oxford OX3 7LD
Telephone: 0865 64811

Riding for the Disabled Association
Avenue R
National Agricultural Centre
Kenilworth
Warwickshire
Telephone: 0203 56107

Scottish Information for the Disabled
Claremont House
18–19 Claremont Crescent
Edinburgh EH7 4QD
Telephone: 031-556 3882

Scottish Sports Association for the Disabled
14 Gordon Court
Dalcaverhouse
Dundee DD4 9DL

Sexual Problems for the Disabled
49 Victoria Street
London SW1

The Disabled Living Foundation
380–384 Harrow Road
London W9 2HU
Telephone: 01-289 6111

The Royal Association for Disability and
Rehabilitation (RADAR)
25 Mortimer Street
London W1N 8AB
Telephone: 01-637 5400

Documentation and retrieval aids

Communication Aids Centre
Boulton Road
West Bromwich
West Midlands
Telephone: 021-553 0908

Possum Users Association
27 Thames House
140 Battersea Park Road
London SW11
Telephone: 01-622 3738

The National Listening Library—Talking
Books
12 Lant Street
London SE1 1QR
Telephone: 01-407 9417

Geriatric amenities and societies

Age Concern England
Bernard Sunley House
60 Pitcairn Road
Mitcham
Surrey CR4 3LL
Telephone: 01-640 5431

British Association for Service to the Elderly
3 Keele Farm House
Keele
Newcastle-under-Lyme
Staffs ST5 5AR
Telephone: 0782 627280

Friends of the Elderly & Gentlefolk
42 Ebury Street
London SW1W 0LZ
Telephone: 01-730 8263

Help the Aged
1 Seckforde Street
London EC1
Telephone: 01-253 0253

National associations & charities

Action for the Research into Multiple
Sclerosis
71 Grays Inn Road
London WC1X 8TR
Telephone: 01-961 4911

Arthritis Care
6 Grosvenor Crescent
London SW1X 7ER
Telephone: 01-235 0902

Arthritis & Rheumatism Council for
Research
41 Eagle Street
London WC1R 4AR
Telephone: 01-405 8572

Asthma Research Council
St Thomas's Hospital
Lambeth Palace Road
London SE1 7EH
Telephone: 01-582 8744

Association to Combat Huntingdon's Chorea
Borough House
34a Station Road
Hinkley
Leics
Telephone: 0455 615558

Association for Spina Bifida &
Hydrocephalus
Tavistock House North
Tavistock Square
London WC1H 9HJ
Telephone: 01-388 1382

British Home & Hospital for the Incurables
Crown Lane
London SW16 3JB
Telephone: 01-670 8261

British Tinnitus Association
105 Gower Street
London WC1 6A4

British Polio Fellowship
Bell Close
West End Road
Ruislip HA4 6LP
Telephone: 08956 75515

Help for Health: Patient Care Information
Service
Wessex Regional Library Unit
Southampton General Hospital
Southampton SO9 4XY
Telephone: 0703 777222, Ext. 3753

Ileostomy Association
Amblehurst House
Chobham
Woking
Surrey GU24 8PZ
Telephone: 099 05 8277

MENCAP
Society for Mentally Handicapped Children
& Adults
123 Golden Lane
London EC1Y 0RT
Telephone: 01-253 9433

Muscular Dystrophy Group
Nattrass House
35 Macaulay Road
London SW4 0QP
Telephone: 01-720 8055

National Ankylosing Spondylitis Society
6 Grosvenor Crescent
London SW1X 7ER
Telephone: 01-235 9585

National Association for Mental Health
(MIND)
22 Harley Street
London W1
Telephone: 01-637 0741

National Association for Patient
Participation in General Practice
28 Heol y Deryn
Glyncorrwg
Port Talbot
West Glamorgan
Telephone: 0639 850 604

Parkinson's Disease Society
36 Portland Place
London W1N 3DG
Telephone: 01-323 1174

Patients Association
11 Dartmouth Street
London SW1H 9BN
Telephone: 01-222 4992

Psoriasis Association
7 Milton Street
Northampton NN2 7JG
Telephone: 0604 711129

Spinal Injuries Association
5 Crowndale Road
London NW1 1TU
Telephone: 01-388 6840

The Chest, Heart & Stroke Association
Tavistock House North
Tavistock Square
London WC1H 9JE
Telephone: 01-387 3012

The Colostomy Welfare Group
38–39 Eccleston Square
2nd Floor
London SW1V 1PB
Telephone: 01-828 5175

The Multiple Sclerosis Society of Great
Britain
286 Munster Road
Fulham
London SW6 6AP
Telephone: 01-381 4022

The National Autistic Society
276 Willesden Lane
London NW2 5RB
Telephone: 01-451 3844/5

The Royal Institute for the Blind
224 Great Portland Street
London W1N 6AA
Telephone: 01-388 1266

The Royal Institute for the Deaf
105 Gower Street
London WC1E 6AH
Telephone: 01-387 8033

The Samaritans
17 Uxbridge Road
Slough SL1 1SN
Telephone: 0753 32713/4

Voluntary Service Overseas
9 Belgrave Square
London SW8X 9PW
Telephone: 01-235 5191

Weight Watchers UK Ltd
11 Fairacres
Bedworth Road
Windsor
Berks
Telephone: Windsor 567751

Widows

Cruse for Widows
Cruse House
126 Sheen
Richmond
Surrey
Telephone: 01-940 4818

National Association for Widows
Chell Road
Stafford ST16 2QA
Telephone: 0785 45465

Sports organisations

Athletics
Amateur Athletics Association
Francis House
Francis Street
London SW1P 1DL
Telephone: 01-828 9129

British Amateur Athletics Board
Francis House
Francis Street
London SW1P 1DL
Telephone: 01-828 9326

Badminton
Badminton Association of England
Bracknell Road
Loughton Lodge
Milton Keynes
Bucks
Telephone: 0908 568822

Cycling
British Cycling Federation
Upper Woburn Place
London WC1 0GE
Telephone: 01-387 9320

Fencing
Amateur Fencing Association
The de Beaumont Centre
Denham Road
West Kensington W14 9SP
Telephone: 01-385 7442

Gymnastics
British Amateur Gymnastics Association
5 High Street
Slough
Berks SL1 1DH
Telephone: Slough 32763

Judo
British Judo Association
16 Upper Woburn Place
London
Telephone: 01-387 9340

Lawn tennis
Lawn Tennis Association
Barons Court
West Kensington
London W14 9EG
Telephone: 01-385 2366

Modern Pentathlon
1a Godstone Road
Purley
Surrey CR2 2DH
Telephone: 01-668 7855/7851

Movement and dance
Keep Fit Association
16 Upper Woburn Place
London WC
Telephone: 01-387 4349

Raquetball
British Raquetball Association
c/o Cresta Raquets Ltd
Blandford Heights
Blandford
Dorset DT11 7TE
Telephone: 0258 5466

Rambling
The Ramblers Association
1–5 Wandsworth Road
London SW8 1LJ
Telephone: 01-582 6878

Ski-ing
British Ski Federation
118 Eaton Square
London SW1W 9AF
Telephone: 01-235 8227

Squash rackets
Squash Rackets Association
Francis House
Francis Street
London SW1P 1DE
Telephone: 01-828 3064

Womens Squash Rackets Association
345 Upper Richmond Road West
Sheen
London SW14 8QN
Telephone: 01-876 6219

Swimming
Amateur Swimming Association
Harold Fern House
Derby Square
Loughborough
Leics LE11 0AL
Telephone: Loughborough 230431

Table tennis
English Table Tennis Association
21 Claremont
Hastings
East Sussex TN34 1HA
Telephone: Hastings 433121

Tennis and rackets
Tennis and Rackets Association
c/o The Queen's Club
Palliser Road
London W14 9EQ
Telephone: 01-381 4746

Trampolining
British Trampoline Federation Ltd
152a College Road
Harrow, Middlesex

Underwater swimming
British Sub-Aqua Club
16 Upper Woburn Place
London WC1H 0QW
Telephone: 01-387 9302

Volleyball
English Volleyball Association
128 Melton Road
West Bridgford
Nottingham NG2 6EP
Telephone: Nottingham 816324

Water ski-ing
British Water Ski Federation
16 Upper Woburn Place
London WC1H 0QL
Telephone: 01-387 9371

Weight lifting
British Amateur Weight Lifting Association
3 Iffley Turn
Oxford
Telephone: Oxford 778319

Yoga
British Wheel of Yoga
88 Leckhampton Road
Cheltenham, Glos
Telephone: Cheltenham 24889

Sports medicine

Association of Chartered Physiotherapists in
Sports Medicine
14 Bedford Row
London WC1
Telephone: 01-242 1941

Central Council for Physical Recreation
70 Brompton Road
London SW3
Telephone: 01-584 6651/3310

Central Council for Physical Recreation
Francis House
Francis Street
London SW1
Telephone: 01-828 3163

British Association of Sport and Medicine
Half Moon Place
Burwash Road
Heathfield TN21 8QN
Telephone: 04352 4607

British Association of Trauma in Sport
110 Harley Street
London W1
Telephone: 01-486 2494

Sports Council
60 Upper Woburn Place
London WC1
Telephone: 01-388 1277

Business and office information: Useful sources

Accountants

England
Institute of Chartered Accountants
PO Box 433
Moorgate Place
London EC2P 2BJ
Telephone: 01-628 7060

Scotland
27 Queen Street
Edinburgh EH2 1LA

The Association of Certified Accountants
29 Lincoln Inn Fields
London WC2A 3EE

The British Association of Accountants and Auditors
Stamford House
2 Chiswick High Road
London W4 1SU

Solicitors
Law Society
113 Chancery Lane
London WC2A 1PL
Telephone: 01-242 1222

Buildings and surveyors

The Building Societies Association
14 Park Street
London W1Y 4AL
Telephone: 01-629 0515

34 Park Street
London W1Y 3PS
Telephone: 01-629 6712

The Land Registry
Lincoln Inn Fields
London WC2A 3PH
Telephone: 01-405 3488

Institute of Chartered Surveyors
George Street
London

Business organisations

Alliance of Small Firms & Self Employed People
42 Vine Road
East Molesey
Surrey KT8 9LF
Telephone: 01-979 2293

279 Church Road
London SE19 2QQ
Telephone: 01-653 4798

Association of Independent Business
Europe House
World Trade Centre
London E1 9AA
Telephone: 01-481 8669

British Institute of Management
Small Firms Information Service
Management House
Parker Street
London WC2B 5PT
Telephone: 01-405 3456

British Insurance Association
Aldermary House
Queen Street
London EC4 4JD
Telephone: 01-248 4477

Business in the Community
227a City Road
London EC1V 1JU
Telephone: 01-235 3716

25 St Andrew's Square
Edinburgh EH1 2AF
Telephone: 031 556 9761

Companies Registration Office
Companies House
55 City Road
London EC1

Companies House
Crown Way
Maindy
Cardiff CF4 3UZ

The Scottish Registrar of Companies
102 George Street
Edinburgh EH2 3DJ

Design Council
28 Haymarket
London SW1 4DG
Telephone: 01-839 8000

Equipment Leasing Association
18 Upper Grosvenor Street
London W1X 9PR
Telephone: 01-491 2783

Finance Houses Association
18 Upper Grosvenor Street
London W1X 9PB
Telephone: 01-491 2783

Institute of Directors
116 Pall Mall
London SW1 5ED
Telephone: 01-839 1233

Institute of Small Businesses
Tower Suite
1 Whitehall Place
London SW1A 2HD
Telephone: 01-930 5577

National Federation of Self Employed and
Small Businesses
32 St Anne's Road West
Lytham St Anne's
Lancashire FY8 1NY
Telephone: 0253 720911
London office: 01-439 8546

Computers

British Medical Data Systems
Primary Care Division
Paddington House
Town Centre
Basingstoke
Hampshire RG21 1LJ
Telephone: 0256 57100

The Data Protection Registrar
Springfield House
Water Lane
Wilmslow
Cheshire SK9 5AX
Telephone: (0625) 535 777/535 711

Fire precautions

Chubb Fire Security Ltd
Head Office
Pyrene House
Sunbury-on-Thames
Middlesex
Telephone: Sunbury-on-Thames 85588

136 Staines Road
Feltham
Middlesex TW14 0JT
Telephone: 01-890 1666

Insurance brokers

The British Insurance Brokers Association
(BIBA)
Fountain House
130 Fenchurch Street
London EC3M 5DJ
Telephone: 01-623 9043

The Insurance Brokers Registration Council
15 St Helens Place
London EC3A 6DS

Insurance companies

Abbey Life Assurance Co
Abbey Life House
1 St Paul's Churchyard
London EC4
Telephone: 01-248 9111

Frizzell Bolton Corder
Bolton House
56–58 Parkstone Road
Poole
Dorset BH15 2PH
Telephone: 0202 671117

Hambro Life
9 Sackville Street
London W1
Telephone: 01-434 3211

Permanent Insurance Co Ltd
7–10 Chandos Street
Cavendish Square
London W1A 2LN
Telephone: 01-636 1686

Sun Alliance & London Insurance Group
1 Bartholomew Lane
London EC2
Telephone: 01-588 2345

The Norwich Union
Surrey Street
Norwich NR1 3JW

51 Fenchurch Street
London EC3
Telephone: 01-623 7733
           01-623 2573

The Royal National Pension Fund for
Nurses
Burdett House
15 Buckingham Street
London WC2N 6ED
Telephone: 01-839 6785

Leasing companies

Atlantic Medical Ltd
Atlantic House
Red Lion Court
London EC4A 3EB
Telephone: 01-583 9481

Station House
Stamford New Road
Altrincham
Cheshire
Telephone: 061 941 6333

Lease Management Services Ltd
Buckland House
Claremont Lane
Esher
Surrey KT10 8BR
Telephone: 0372 67711

Lion Chambers
170 Hope Street
Glasgow G2 2TU
Telephone: 041 333 0710

Medenta Services Ltd
276 High Street
Guildford GU1 3JL
Telephone: 0483 39164

62 Broughton Street
Edinburgh EH1 3SA
Telephone: 031 557 1554

Hamilton House
80 Stokes Croft
Bristol BS1 3QW
Telephone: 0272 42220

Motoring organisations

The Automobile Association
Head Office
PO Box 50
Basingstoke
Hants RG21 2ED
Telephone: 0256 24872

The Royal Automobile Club
149 Pall Mall
London SW1
Telephone: 01-839 7050

Professional nameplates

Abbey Craftsmen Ltd
4 Park Works
Kingsley
Bordon
Hants
Telephone: 042 03 2091

Telephone sales centres

British Telecom
Manhattan House
High Street
Crowthorne
Berks RG11 1BR
Telephone: 730 0899

Cellcall Ltd
5 St Botolph Street
London EC3A 7DT
Telephone: 01-283 1122

Cellnet Accredited Retailers
Dept CSI Admail 2000
London NW9 5AL
Telephone: 01-22 0200

Racal Vodac Ltd
Freepost
Newbury RG13 1DR
Telephone: Freefone 100

Northern Ireland

As for rest of U.K.

Government health organisations

Eastern Health & Social Services Board
Londonderry House
Chichester Street
Belfast 1

Northern Health & Social Services Board
County Hall
Galgorm Road
Ballymena
Co. Antrim

Southern Health & Social Services Board
20 Seagoe Industrial Area
Portadown
Co. Armagh

Western Health & Social Services Board
15 Gransha Park
Campsie
Co. Londonderry

Professional organisations

As for rest of U.K.

British Medical Association
British Dental Association
Chartered Society of Physiotherapy
OCPPP
Royal College of Nursing
and all other British Medical professional
bodies

Medical insurance

As for rest of U.K.

Taxation offices

Inland Revenue
Controller for Northern Ireland
Windsor House
Bedford Street
Belfast 1

Main banks

Allied Irish Banks Ltd
14 Donegall Square East
Belfast 1

Bank of Ireland
54 Donegall Place
Belfast 1

Northern Bank Ltd
Donegall Square West
Belfast 1

Trustee Savings Bank of Northern Ireland
4 Queens Square
Belfast

Ulster Bank Ltd
47 Donegall Place
Belfast BT1 5AU

Private hospitals & clinics

Ulster Independent Clinic
Stranmillis Road
Belfast 9

Herron Clinic
Royal Victoria Hospital
Belfast 12

Medical bookshops

William Mullan and Son Ltd
12 Donegall Place
Belfast

University Bookshop
91 University Road
Belfast

Other sources of useful information

Local Enterprise Development Unit
Linenhall Street
Belfast

215

United States of America

The education, taxation and licensing requirements for each State vary and this Appendix is only intended as a general guide. It is strongly recommended that you contact the Social Security Administration for Government programmes. Ask your local office for the Social Security and Medicare Fact Sheet and the Medicare Handbook. Also check with the official professional organisation for current details.

Government health organisations

American Health Care Association
1200 15th Street
Northwest
Washington DC 20005
Telephone: (202) 833 2050

American Health Planning Association
110 Vermont Avenue NW
Suite 950
Washington DC 20005
Telephone: (202) 861 1200

American Public Health Association
1015 15th Street NW
Washington DC 2005
Telephone: (202) 789 5600

American Social Health Association
260 Sheridan Avenue
Suite 307
Palo Alto
California 94306
Telephone: (415) 321 5134

Bureau of National Affairs Inc.
Washington DC 20037

Department of Health & Human Services
Health Care Financing Administration
Baltimore
Maryland 21235

Department of Health & Human Services
Hubert Humphrey Building
200 Independence Avenue SW
Washington 20201
Telephone: (202) 245 6727

National Association of Community Health Centres
1626 1st Street NW
Suite 420
Washington DC 20006
Telephone: (202) 833 9280

National Health Council
70 West 49th Street
New York 10018
Telephone: (212) 869 8100

National Health Council
1700 K Street NW
Washington DC 20006
Telephone: (202) 785 3913

State medical associations

Alabama
Medical Association of the State of Alabama
19 S. Jackson St
PO Box 1900-C
Montgomery AL 36197
Telephone: (205) 263 6441

Alaska
Alaska State Medical Association
1135 W. Eighth Ave
Suite 6
Anchorage AK 99501
Telephone: (907) 277 6891

Arizona
Arizona Medical Association Inc
810 W. Bethany Home Road
Phoenix AZ 85013
Telephone: (602) 246 8901

Arkansas
Arkansas Medical Society
214 N. Twelfth Street
Box 1208
Fort Smith AR 72902
Telephone: (501) 782 8218

California
California Medical Association
731 Market St
San Francisco CA 94103
Telephone: (415) 777 2000

Colorado
Colorado Medical Society
1601 E. Nineteenth Ave
Denver CO 80218
Telephone: (303) 861 1221

Connecticut
Connecticut State Medical Society
160 St Ronan St
New Haven CT 06511
Telephone: (203) 865 0587

Delaware
Medical Society of Delaware
1925 Lovering Ave
Wilmington DE 19806
Telephone: (302) 658 7596

District of Columbia
Medical Society of District of Columbia
2007 Eye St NW
Washington DC 20006
Telephone: (202) 223 2230

Florida
Florida Medical Association Inc
PO Box 2411
760 Riverside Ave
Jacksonville FL 32203
Telephone: (904) 356 1571

Georgia
Medical Association of Georgia
938 Peachtree St
NE. Atlanta GA 30309
Telephone: (404) 876 7535

Hawaii
Hawaii Medical Association
320 Ward Ave
Suite 200
Honolulu HI 96814
Telephone: (808) 536 7702

Idaho
Idaho Medical Association
PO Box 2668
407 W. Bannock St
Boise ID 83701
Telephone: (208) 344 7888

Illinois
Illinois State Medical Society
55 E. Monroe
Suite 3510
Chicago IL 60603
Telephone: (312) 782 1654

Indiana
Indiana State Medical Association
3935 N. Meridian
Indianapolis IN 46208
Telephone: (317) 925 7545

Iowa
Iowa Medical Society
1001 Grand Ave
West Des Moines IA 50265
Telephone: (515) 223 1401

Kansas
Kansas Medical Society
1300 Topeka Boulevard
Topeka KS 66612
Telephone: (913) 235 2383

Kentucky
Kentucky Medical Association
3532 Ephraim McDowell Dr
Louisville KY 40205
Telephone: (502) 459 9790

Louisiana
Louisiana State Medical Society
1700 Josephine St
New Orleans LA 70113
Telephone: (504) 561 1033

Maine
Maine Medical Association
524 Western Ave
Augusta ME 04330
Telephone: (203) 622 3374

Maryland
Medical & Chirurgical Faculty of Maryland
1211 Cathedral St
Baltimore MD 21201
Telephone: (301) 539 0872

Massachusetts
Massachusetts Medical Society
22 Fenway
Boston MA 02215
Telephone: (617) 536 8812

Michigan
Michigan State Medical Society
PO Box 950
120 W. Saginaw
East Lansing MI 48823
Telephone: (517) 337 1351

Minnesota
Minnesota Medical Association
Health Associations Center
2221 University Ave SE
Suite 4000
Minneapolis MN 55414
Telephone: (612) 378 1875

Mississippi
Mississippi State Medical Association
735 Riverside Dr
PO Box 5229
Jackson MS 39216
Telephone: (601) 354 5433

Missouri
Missouri State Medical Association
PO Box 1028
113 Madison St
Jefferson City MO 65101
Telephone: (314) 636 5151

Montana
Montana Medical Association
2021 Eleventh Ave
Suite 12
Helena MT 59601
Telephone: (406) 443 4000

Nebraska
Nebraska Medical Association
1512 First National Bank Bldg
Lincoln NE 68508
Telephone: (402) 432 7585

Nevada
Nevada State Medical Association
3660 Baker Ln
Reno NV 89509
Telephone: (702) 825 6788

New Hampshire
New Hampshire Medical Society
4 Park St
Concord NH 03301
Telephone: (603) 224 1909

New Jersey
Medical Society of New Jersey
2 Princess Rd
Lawrenceville NJ 08648
Telephone: (609) 896 1766

New Mexico
New Mexico Medical Society
PO Box 9366
2650 Yale Boulevard SE
Albuquerque NM 87106
Telephone: (505) 247 0539

New York
Medical Society of the State of New York
420 Lakeville Rd
Lake Success NY 11040
Telephone: (516) 488 6100

North Carolina
North Carolina Medical Society
222 N. Person St
PO Box 27167
Raleigh NC 27611
Telephone: (919) 833 3836

North Dakota
North Dakota Medical Association
PO Box 1198
810 E. Roffer Ave
Bismarck ND 58501
Telephone: (701) 223 9475

Ohio
Ohio State Medical Association
600 S. High St
Columbus OH 43215
Telephone: (614) 228 6971

Oklahoma
Oklahoma State Medical Association
601 NW Expressway
Oklahoma City OK 73118
Telephone: (405) 843 9571

Oregon
Oregon Medical Association
5210 Corbett St
SW. Portland OR 97201
Telephone: (503) 226 1555

Pennsylvania
Pennsylvania Medical Society
PO Box 301
20 Erford Rd
Lemoyne PA 17043
Telephone: (717) 763 7151

Rhode Island
Rhode Island Medical Society
Providence Medical Association
106 Francis St
Providence RI 02903
Telephone: (401) 331 3207

South Carolina
South Carolina Medical Association
3325 Medical Park Rd
Box 11188
Columbia SC 29211
Telephone: (803) 252 6311

South Dakota
South Dakota State Medical Association
608 West Ave North
Sioux Falls SD 57104
Telephone: (605) 336 1965

Tennessee
Tennessee Medical Assocation
112 Louise Ave
Nashville TN 37203
Telephone: (615) 327 1451

Texas
Texas Medical Association
1801 N. Lamar Boulevard
Austin TX 78701
Telephone: (512) 447 6704

Utah
Utah State Medical Association
540 Fifth St South
Salt Lake City UT 84102
Telephone: (801) 355 7477

Vermont
Vermont State Medical Society
136 Main St
Montpelier VT 05602
Telephone: (802) 223 7898

Virginia
Medical Society of Virginia
4205 Dover Rd
Richmond VA 23221
Telephone: (804) 353 2721

Washington
Washington State Medical Association
2033 Sixth Ave
Seattle WA 98121
Telephone: (206) 623 4801

West Virginia
West Virginia State Medical Association
Charleston National Plaza
PO Box 1031
Charleston WV 25324
Telephone: (304) 346 0551

Wisconsin
State Medical Society of Wisconsin
330 E. Lakeside St
Box 1109
Madison WI 53701
Telephone: (608) 257 6781

Wyoming
Wyoming Medical Society
1920 Evans St
PO Drawer 4009
Cheyenne WY 82001
Telephone: (307) 635 2424

Professional organisations

Aerospace Medical Association
Washington National Airport
Washington DC 20001
Telephone: (703) 892 2240

American Academy of Family Physicians
1740 W. Ninety-Second Street
Kansas City MO 64114

600 Maryland Avenue SW
Suite 770
Washington DC 20024
Telephone: (202) 488 7448

American Academy of Orthopaedic
Surgeons
2010 Massachusetts Avenue NW
Suite 600
Washington DC 20815
Telephone: 652 0905

American Academy of Orthotists &
Prosthetists
717 Pendleton Street
Alexandra, Virginia 22314
Telephone: (703) 836 7118

American Academy of Pediatrics
1300 North 17th Street
Suite 350
Arlington, Virginia 22209
Telephone: (703) 525 9560

American Association of Colleges of Nursing
11 Dupont Circle NW
Suite 430
Washington DC 20036
Telephone: (202) 332 1917

American Association of Colleges of
Osteopathic Medicine
6110 Executive Boulevard
Suite 405
Rockville, Maryland 20852
Telephone: (301) 468 0990

American Association of Colleges of
Pharmacy
4630 Montgomery Avenue
Suite 201
Bethesda, Maryland 20814
Telephone: (301) 654 0960

American Association of Colleges of
Podiatric Medicine
6110 Executive Boulevard
Suite 204
Rockville
Maryland 20852
Telephone: (301) 984 9350

American Association of Hospital
Consultants
1235 Jefferson Davis Highway
Suite 602
Arlington
Virginia 22202
Telephone: (703) 979 3180

American Dental Association
211 East Chicago Avenue
Chicago
Illinois 60611
Telephone: (312) 440 2500

American Medical Association
535 North Dearborn Street
Chicago
Illinois 60611
Telephone: (312) 751 6000

American Nurses Association
2420 Pershing Road
Kansas City MO 64108
Telephone: (816) 474 5720

American Occupational Therapy Association
1383 Pickard Drive
Rockville
Maryland 20850
Telephone: (301) 948 9626

American Osteopathic Association
122 C. Street NW
Suite 875
Washington DC 20001
Telephone: (202) 783 3434

American Physical Therapy Association
1111 North Fairfax Street
Alexandria
Virginia 22314
Telephone: (703) 684 2782

American Podiatry Association
20 Chevy Chase Circle NW
Washington 20015
Telephone: (202) 537 4900

American Psychiatric Association
1400 K. Street NW
Washington DC 20005
Telephone: (202) 682 6000

American Speech Language Hearing
Association
10801 Rockville Pike
Rockville
Maryland 20852
Telephone: (301) 897 5700

Medical insurance

National organisations

Health Insurance Association of America
1850 K Street
Northwest
Washington DC 20006

National Association of Insurance
Commissioners (NAIC)
633 W. Wisconsin Avenue
Suite 1015
Milwaukee WI 53203
Telephone: (414) 271 4464

National Council on Compensation
Insurance
One Penn Plaza
New York NY 10001
Telephone: (212) 560 1006

*State Insurance Departments for Specific
Legislation and Regulations affecting Health
Insurance*

State insurance information services

Florida Insurance News Service
PO Box 10088
Tallahassee FL 32302
Telephone: (904) 224-5606

Illinois Insurance Information Service
708 Wrigley Building
400 North Michigan Avenue
Chicago IL 60611
Telephone: (312) 321-0653

Insurance Federation of Pennsylvania
1560 Suburban Station Building
Philadelphia PA 19103
Telephone: (215) 665-0500

Insurance Information Service of Wisconsin
110 East Main Street
Madison WI 53703
Telephone: (608) 257-2011

Insurance Institute of Indiana, Inc.
701 Board of Trade Building
Indianapolis IN 46204
Telephone: (317) 635-2328

Kansas Association of Property & Casualty
Insurance Companies
610 1st National Bank Towers
Topeka KS 66603

Michigan Association of Insurance
Companies
802 Capitol Savings and Loan Building
Lansing MI 48933
Telephone: (517) 482-1643

Minnesota Insurance Information Center
1320 Soo Line Building
Minneapolis MN 55402
Telephone: (612) 339-9273

New Jersey Insurance News Service
971 Stuyvesant Avenue
Union NJ 07083
Telephone: (201) 339-9273

North Carolina Insurance News Service
PO Box 11526
Charlotte NC 28209
Telephone: (704) 372-8775

Ohio Insurance Institute
PO Box 632
Columbus OH 43216
Telephone: (614) 228-1593

South Carolina Insurance News Service
708 Columbia Building
1200 Gervais Street
Columbia SC 29201
Telephone: (803) 252-2355

Southwestern Insurance Information
Service
8705 Shoal Creek Boulevard
Suite 212
Austin TX 78758
Telephone: (512) 458-8214

Texas Insurance Information Center
1011 Congress Avenue
Suite 501
Austin TX 78701
Telephone: (512) 476-7025

Washington Insurance Council
1218 Third Avenue
Room 2203
Seattle WA 98101
Telephone: (206) 624-3330

Western Insurance Information Service
1450 North Tustin Avenue
Suite 124
Santa Ana CA 92701
Telephone: (714) 558-1052

State insurance departments

Alabama: Commissioner of Insurance
64 North Union Street
Montgomery AL 36130
Telephone: (205) 832-6140

Alaska: Director of Insurance
Room 410
Goldstein Building
Pouch D
Juneau AK 99811
Telephone: (907) 465-2515

Arizona: Director of Insurance
1601 West Jefferson
Phoenix AZ 85007
Telephone: (602) 255-5400

Arkansas: Insurance Commissioner
12th & University Avenue
Little Rock AR 72204
Telephone: (501) 371-1325

California: Insurance Commissioner
100 Van Ness
San Francisco CA 94102
Telephone: (415) 557-1126

Colorado: Commissioner of Insurance
106 State Office Building
Denver CO 80203
Telephone: (303) 866-3201

Connecticut: Insurance Commissioner
425 State Office Building
Hartford CT 06115
Telephone: (203) 566-5275

Delaware: Insurance Commissioner
21 The Green
Dover DE 19901
Telephone: (302) 736-4251

District of Columbia: Superintendent of
Insurance
614 H Street Northwest
Suite 512
Washington DC 20001
Telephone: (202) 727-1273

Florida: Insurance Commissioner
State Capitol
Tallahassee FL 32304
Telephone: (904) 488-3440

Georgia: Insurance Commissioner
238 State Capitol
Atlanta GA 30334
Telephone: (404) 656-2056

Hawaii: Insurance Commissioner
PO Box 3614
Honolulu HI 96811
Telephone: (808) 548-7505

Idaho: Director of Insurance
700 West State Street
Boise ID 83720
Telephone: (208) 334-2250

Illinois: Director of Insurance
320 West Washington
Springfield IL 62767
Telephone: (217) 785-5516

Indiana: Commissioner of Insurance
509 State Office Building
Indianapolis IN 46204
Telephone: (317) 232-2386

Iowa: Director of Insurance
State Office Building
Des Moines, Iowa 50319
Telephone: (515) 281-5705

Kansas: Commissioner of Insurance
State Office Building
Topeka KS 66612
Telephone: (913) 296-3071

Kentucky: Insurance Commissioner
151 Elkhorn Court
Frankfort KY 40601
Telephone: (502) 564-3630

Louisiana: Commissioner of Insurance
PO Box 44214
Capitol Station
Baton Rouge LA 70804
Telephone: (504) 342-5328

Maine: Superintendent of Insurance
Department of Business Regulation
State House Station #34
Augusta ME 04333
Telephone: (207) 289-3101

Maryland: Insurance Commissioner
One South Calvert Building
Baltimore MD 21202
Telephone: (301) 659-6300

Massachusetts: Commissioner of Insurance
100 Cambridge Street
Boston MA 02202
Telephone: (617) 727-3333

Michigan: Commissioner of Insurance
PO Box 30220
Lansing MI 48909
Telephone: (517) 373-0220

Minnesota: Commissioner of Insurance
Metro Square Building
St Paul MN 55101
Telephone: (612) 296-6907

Mississippi: Commissioner of Insurance
PO Box 2306
Jackson MS 39205
Telephone: (601) 354-7711

Missouri: Director of Insurance
PO Box 690
Jefferson City MO 65102
Telephone: (314) 751-4126

Montana: Commissioner of Insurance
Mitchel Building
PO Box 4009
Helena MT 59604
Telephone: (406) 449-2996

Nebraska: Director of Insurance
301 Centennial Mall South
Lincoln NE 68509
Telephone: (402) 471-2201

Nevada: Insurance Commissioner
201 South Fall Street
Carson City NV 89701
Telephone: (702) 885-4270

New Hampshire: Insurance Commissioner
169 Manchester Street
Concord NH 03301
Telephone: (603) 271-2261

New Jersey: Commissioner of Insurance
201 East State Street
Trenton NJ 08625
Telephone: (609) 292-5363

New Mexico: Superintendent of Insurance
PO Drawer 1269
Santa Fe NM 87501
Telephone: (505) 827-2451

New York: Superintendent of Insurance
Two World Trade Center
New York NY 10047
Telephone: (212) 488-4124

North Carolina: Commissioner of Insurance
PO Box 26387
Raleigh NC 27611
Telephone: (919) 733-7343

North Dakota: Commissioner of Insurance
Capitol Building
Fifth Floor
Bismarck ND 58501
Telephone: (701) 224-2444

Ohio: Director of Insurance
2100 Stella Court
Columbus OH 43215
Telephone: (614) 466-2691

Oklahoma: Insurance Commissioner
408 Will Rogers Memorial Building
Oklahoma City OK 73105
Telephone: (405) 521-2828

Oregon: Insurance Commissioner
158 12th Street, Northeast
Salem OR 97310
Telephone: (503) 378-4271

Pennsylvania: Insurance Commissioner
13th Floor
Strawberry Square
Harrisburg PA 17120
Telephone: (717) 787-5173

Puerto Rico: Commissioner of Insurance
PO Box 3508
San Juan PR 00904
Telephone: (809) 722-0141

Rhode Island: Insurance Commissioner
100 North Main Street
Providence RI 02903
Telephone: (401) 277-2223

South Carolina: Insurance Commissioner
2711 Middleburg Drive
Columbia SC 29204
Telephone: (803) 758-2185

South Dakota: Commissioner of Insurance
Insurance Building
Pierre SD 57501
Telephone: (605) 773-3564

Tennessee: Commissioner of Insurance
114 State Office Building
Nashville TN 37219
Telephone: (615) 741-2241

Texas: Commissioner of Insurance
1110 San Jacinto Boulevard
Austin TX 78786
Telephone: (512) 475-2273

Utah: Commissioner of Insurance
326 South Fifth East
Salt Lake City UT 84102
Telephone: (801) 533-5611

Vermont: Commissioner of Insurance
State Office Building
Montpelier VT 05602
Telephone: (802) 828-3301

Virginia: Commissioner of Insurance
PO Box 1157
Richmond VA 23209
Telephone: (804) 786-3741

Washington: Insurance Commissioner
Insurance Building
Olympia WA 98504
Telephone: (206) 753-7301

West Virginia: Insurance Commissioner
2100 Washington Street East
Charleston WV 25305
Telephone: (302) 348-3386

Wisconsin: Commissioner of Insurance
PO Box 7873
Madison WI 53707
Telephone: (608) 266-3585

Wyoming: Insurance Commissioner
2424 Pioneer Street
Cheyenne WY 82002
Telephone: (307) 777-7310

Health insurance companies

Aetna Life & Casualty Company
151 Farmington Avenue
Hartford CT 06115
Telephone: (203) 273 0123

Continental Assurance Company
CNA Plaza
Chicago
Illinois 60685
Telephone: (312) 822 5000

Connecticut General Life Insurance
Company
900 Cottage Grove Road
Bloomfield CT
Mailing address: Hartford CT 06152
Telephone: (203) 726 6000

Equitable Life of New York
1285 Avenue of the Americas
New York NY 10019
Telephone: (212) 554 1234

Lincoln National Life Insurance Company
1300 South Clinton Street
Fort Wayne IN 46801
Telephone: (219) 424 5421

Metropolitan Life Insurance Company
One Madison Avenue
New York NY 10010
Telephone: (212) 578 2211

Mutual of Omaha
Dodge at 33rd Street
Omaha NE 68131
Telephone: (402) 342 7600

Occidental Life Insurance
Occidental Center
1150 South Olive
Los Angeles CA 90015
Telephone: (213) 742 2111

Prudential Insurance Company of America
Prudential Plaza
Newark NJ 07101
Telephone: (201) 877 6000

Travelers Insurance Company
One Tower Square
Hartford CT 06115
Telephone: (203) 277 0111

*Blue Cross and Blue Shield Associations &
Plans*

1709 New York Avenue NW
Suite 303
Washington DC 20006
Telephone: (202) 783 6222

Alabama
Blue Cross & Blue Shield of Alabama
PO Box 995
450 Richerchase Parkway
Birmingham AL 35298

Alaska
See Blue Cross of Washington & Alaska

Arizona
Blue Cross & Blue Shield of Arizona Inc.
PO Box 13466
321 W. Indian School Road
Phoenix AZ 85013

Arkansas
Arkansas Blue Cross & Blue Shield Inc.
PO Box 2181
601 Gaines St
Little Rock AR 72203

California
Blue Shield of California
PO Box 3637
2 N. Point
San Francisco CA 94119

Blue Cross of Southern California
PO Box 70000
21555 Oxnard St
Van Nuys CA 91470

Blue Cross of Northern California
1950 Franklin St
Oakland CA 94659

Colorado
Blue Cross & Blue Shield of Colorado
700 Broadway
Denver CO 80273

Connecticut
Blue Cross & Blue Shield of Connecticut
Inc.
PO Box 504
370 Bassett Rd
North Haven CT 06473

Delaware
Blue Cross & Blue Shield of Delaware Inc.
PO Box 1991
201 W. Fourteenth St
Wilmington DE 19801

District of Columbia
District of Columbia-Group Hospital Inc.
550 Twelfth St SW
Washington DC 20024

Florida
Blue Cross & Blue Shield of Florida Inc.
PO Box 1798
532 Riverside Avenue
Jacksonville FL 32231

Georgia
Blue Cross & Blue Shield of Georgia/Atlanta
Inc.
PO Box 4445
Atlanta GA 30302

Blue Cross of Georgia/Columbia
PO Box 7368
2357 Warm Springs Road
Columbus GA 31904

Hawaii
Hawaii Medical Service Association
PO Box 860
1504 Kapiolani Boulevard
Honolulu HI 96814

Idaho
Blue Cross of Idaho Health Service Inc.
PO Box 7408
1501 Federal Way
Boise ID 83705

Blue Shield of Idaho
PO Box 1106
1602 Twenty-First Avenue
Lewiston ID 83501

Illinois
Health Care Service Corporation
PO Box 1364
233 N. Michigan Avenue
Chicago ILL 60690

Rockford Blue Cross
(Illinois Hospital & Health Service Inc.)
227 Wyman St
Rockford ILL 61101

Indiana
Blue Cross of Indiana
120 W. Market St
Indianapolis IN 46204

Blue Shield of Indiana
120 W. Market St
Indianapolis IN 46204

Iowa
Blue Cross & Blue Shield of Iowa
636 Grand Avenue
Des Moines IA 50307

Blue Cross of Western Iowa & South Dakota
PO Box 1677
Hamilton Boulevard & 1–29
Sioux City IA 51102

Kansas
Blue Cross & Blue Shield of Kansas
PO Box 239
1133 Topeka Avenue
Topeka KS 66601

Kentucky
Blue Cross & Blue Shield of Kentucky Inc.
9901 Linn Station Rd
Louisville KY 40223

Louisiana
Blue Cross of Louisiana
PO Box 15699
10225 Florida Boulevard
Baton Rouge LA 70895

Maine
Blue Cross & Blue Shield of Maine
110 Free St
Portland ME 04101

Maryland
Blue Cross of Maryland Inc.
PO Box 9836
700 E. Joppa Rd
Baltimore MD 21204

Massachusetts
Blue Cross & Blue Shield of Massachusetts
Inc.
100 Summer St
Boston MA 02106

Michigan
Blue Cross & Blue Shield of Michigan
600 Lafayette E.
Detroit MI 48226

Minnesota
Blue Cross & Blue Shield of Minnesota
PO Box 43560
3535 Blue Cross Rd
St Paul MN 55164

Mississippi
Blue Cross & Blue Shield of Mississippi Inc.
PO Box 1043
Lakeland Drive
East at Flynt
Jackson MS 39205

Missouri
Blue Cross Hospital Service Inc. of Missouri
4444 Forest Park Boulevard
St Louis MO 63108

Blue Cross of Kansas City
PO Box 169
3637 Broadway
Kansas City MO 64141

St Louis Blue Shield
(Missouri Medical Service)
4444 Forest Park Boulevard
St Louis MO 63108

Montana
Blue Cross of Montana
PO Box 5004
3360 Tenth Ave South
Great Falls MT 59405

Blue Shield of Montana
(Montana Physician's Service)
Box 4309
404 Fuller Ave
Helena MT 59601

Nebraska
Blue Cross & Blue Shield of Nebraska
PO Box 3248
Main PO Station
Omaha NE 68180

Nevada
Blue Shield of Nevada
PO Box 10330
4600 Kietzke Ln
Reno NV 89502

New Hampshire
New Hampshire-Vermont Health Service
2 Pillsbury St
Concord NH 03301

New Jersey
Hospital Service Plan of New Jersey
PO Box 420
33 Washington St
Newark NJ 07102

Medical-Surgical Plan of New Jersey
33 Washington St
Newark NJ 07102

New Mexico
New Mexico Blue Cross & Blue Shield Inc.
12800 Indian School Rd NE
Albuquerque NM 87112

New York
Blue Cross of Central New York Inc.
PO Box 4809
344 S. Warren St
Syracuse NY 10017

Blue Cross & Blue Shield of Greater New
York
PO Box 345
Grand Central Station
New York NY 10017

Blue Cross of Northeastern New York Inc.
PO Box 8650
1251 New Scotland Rd
Albany NY 12208

Blue Cross of Western New York Inc.
298 Main St
Buffalo NY 14202

Genesee Valley Medical Care Inc.
41 Chestnut St
Rochester NY 14647

Hospital Plan Inc.
5 Hopper St
Utica NY 13501

Hospital Service Corporation of Jefferson
County
Box 570
Stone St
Watertown NY 13601

Medical & Surgical Care Inc.
245 Genesee St
Utica NY 13501

Rochester Hospital Service Corporation
41 Chestnut St
Rochester NY 14647

North Carolina
Blue Cross & Blue Shield of North Carolina
PO Box 2291
5901 Chapel Hill-Durham Boulevard
Durham NC 27702

North Dakota
Blue Cross of North Dakota
4510 Thirteenth Ave SW
Fargo ND 58121

Ohio
Blue Cross in Canton
Box 8590
4150 Belden Village St NW
Canton OH 44718

Blue Cross of Central Ohio
Box 16526
255 E. Main St
Columbus OH 43215

Blue Cross in Eastern Ohio
2400 Market St
Youngstown OH 44507

Blue Cross in Lima
Box 1046
50 Town Sq.
Lima OH 45802

Blue Cross of Northeast Ohio
2066 E. Ninth St
Cleveland OH 44115

Blue Cross of Northwest Ohio
PO Box 943
3737 Sylvania Ave
Toledo OH 43656

Blue Cross in Southwest Ohio
1351 William Howard
Taft Rd
Cincinnati OH 45206

Hospital Care Corporation
1351 William Howard
Taft Rd
Cincinnati OH 45206

Medical Mutual of Cleveland Inc.
2060 E. Ninth St
Cleveland OH 44115

Ohio Medical Indemnity Mutual Corp.
6740 N. Hight St
Worthington OH 43085

Oklahoma
Blue Cross & Blue Shield of Oklahoma
(Group Hospital Service)
PO Box 3283
1215 S. Boulder Ave
Tulsa OK 74119

Oregon
Blue Cross of Oregon
PO Box 1271
100 SW Market St
Portland OR 97201

Pennsylvania
Blue Cross of Greater Philadelphia
1333 Chestnut St
Philadelphia PA 19107

Blue Cross of Lehigh Valley
1221 Hamilton St
Allentown PA 18102

Blue Cross of Northeastern Pennsylvania
70 N. Main St
Wilkes-Barre PA 18711

Blue Cross of Western Pennsylvania
1 Smithfield St
Pittsburgh PA 15222

Capital Blue Cross
100 Pine St
Harrisburg PA 17101

Pennsylvania Blue Shield
Camp Hill PA 17011

Rhode Island
Blue Cross & Blue Shield of Rhode Island
444 Westminster Mall
Providence RU 02901

South Carolina
Blue Cross & Blue Shield of South Carolina
1–20 East at Alpine Rd
Columbia SC 29219

South Dakota
See Iowa

Tennessee
Blue Cross & Blue Shield of Tennessee
801 Pine St
Chattanooga TN 37401
Memphis Hospital Service & Surgical
Association Inc.
PO Box 98
85 N. Danny Thomas Boulevard
Memphis TN 38101

Texas
Group Hospital Service Inc.
PO Box 225730
Main at North Central Expressway
Dallas TX 75201

Utah
Blue Cross & Blue Shield of Utah
PO Box 30270
2455 Parkey's Way
Salt Lake City UT 84130

Vermont
See New Hampshire

Virginia
Blue Cross of Southwestern Virginia
PO Box 13047
3959 Electric Rd SW
Roanoke VA 24045

Blue Cross of Virginia
PO Box 27401
1015 Staples Mill Rd
Richmond VA 23230

Washington
Blue Cross of Washington & Alaska
PO Box 327
15700 Dayton Ave North
Seattle WA 98111

Chelan County Medical Service Corporation
Box 580
707 N. Emerson
Wenatchee WA 98801

King County Medical Blue Shield
Box 21267
1800 Terry Ave
Seattle WA 98101

Medical Service Corporation for Eastern
Washington
PO Box 3048
Terminal Annex
Spokane WA 99202

Pierce County Medical Bureau Inc.
1114 Broadway Plaza
Tacoma WA 98402

Washington Physicians' Service
Fourth & Battery Bldg
Suite 600
2401 Fourth Ave
Seattle WA 98121

West Virginia
Blue Cross Hospital Service Inc.
PO Box 1353
Commerce Sq.
Charleston WV 25325

Blue Cross of Northern West Virginia Inc.
PO Box 7026
Twentieth & Chapline Streets
Wheeling WV 26003

Blue Cross of West Central West Virginia
PO Box 1948
Seventh & Market Streets
Parkersburg WV 26101

Morgantown Medical-Surgical Service Inc.
265 High St
Morgantown WV 26505

Wisconsin
Blue Cross & Blue Shield of Wisconsin
PO Box 2025
401 W. Michigan St
Milwaukee WI 53201

Wyoming
Blue Cross & Blue Shield of Wyoming
PO Box 2266
400 House Ave
Cheyenne WY 82001

Alternative group health insurance

American Association of Foundations for
Medical Care
1900 M Street
Washington DC 20036
Telephone: (202) 466 2628

Group Health Association of America Inc.
1717 Massachusetts Avenue Northwest
Washington DC 20036
Telephone: (202) 483 4012

Private independent hospitals and clinics

American Association for Hospital Planning
1101 Connecticut Avenue NW
Suite 700
Washington DC 20036
Telephone: (202) 857 1162

American Association of Hospital
Consultants
1235 Jefferson Davis Highway
Suite 602
Arlington
Virginia 22202
Telephone: (703) 979 3180

American Hospital Association
444 North Capitol St
Washington DC 20661
Telephone: (202) 638 1100

American Hospital Association
840 North Lake Shore Drive
Chicago ILL 60611
Telephone: (312) 280 6000

American Hospital Supply Corp.
1090 Vermont Avenue NW
Suite 210
Washington DC 20005
Telephone: (202) 842 3445

American Osteopathic Hospital
Association
1025 Vermont Avenue NW
Suite 800
Washington DC 2005
Telephone: (202) 783 5584

American Society of Hospital Pharmacists
4630 Montgomery Avenue
Bethesda
Maryland 20814
Telephone: (301) 657 3000

Federation of American Hospitals
1111 19th Street NW
Suite 402
Washington DC 20036
Telephone: (202) 833 3090

Hospital Financial Management Association
666 North Lake Shore Drive
Chicago ILL 60611
Telephone: (312) 649 5151

National Association of Childrens Hospitals
& Related Institutions
325 First Street
Alexandra
Virginia 22314
Telephone: (703) 684 1355

National Association of Hospital Admitting
Managers
1101 Connecticut Avenue NW
Suite 700
Washington DC 20036
Telephone: (202) 857 1125

National Association for Hospital
Development
8300 Greensboro Drive
Suite 1110
McLean
Virginia 22102
Telephone: (703) 556 9555

National Association of Psychiatric Hospitals
1319 F Street NW
Suite 1000
Washington DC 20003
Telephone: (202) 393 6700

National Association of Public Hospitals
1775 Pennsylvania Avenue NW
Suite 600
Washington DC 20006
Telephone: (202) 628 2721

National Council of Community Hospitals
1000 Thomas Jefferson Street NW
Suite 500
Washington DC 20007
Telephone: (202) 342 7300

Voluntary Hospitals of America
1730 Rhode Island Avenue NW
Suite 801
Washington DC 20036
Telephone: (202) 822 9750

Washington Business Group on Health
922 Pennsylvania Avenue SE
Washington DC 20003
Telephone: (202) 547 6644

Hospital and clinic management

Advanced Health Systems Inc.
2415 S. 2300 West
Salt Lake City UT 84119

American Medical International
6400 Powers Ferry Rd
Atlanta GA 30339

A. E. Brim & Associates
177 NE 102nd Ave
Portland OR 97236

Calumet Memorial Hospital
614 Memorial Dr.
Chilton WI 53014

Carolinas Hospital & Health Services
PO Box 12546
Raleigh NC 27605

Family Health Care Centers
444 N. Michigan Ave
Suite 3650
Chicago IL 60611

Hospital Affiliates International
Western Division
7616 L.B.J. Freeway, S-303
Dallas TX 75251

Hospital Affiliates Management Corp.
Eastern Division
6520 Powers Ferry Rd
S-300 Atlanta GA 30339

Hospital Affiliates Management Corp.
Western Division
6225 U.S. Highway 290 E.
Suite 201
Austin TX 78723

Hospital Corporation of America
PO Box 550
1 Park Plaza
Nashville TN 37202

Hospital Management Associates
2180 W. First St
Suite 510
Fort Myers FL 33901

Humana Corp.
PO Box 1430
Louisville KY 40201

Jackson & Coker
4488 N. Shallowford Rd
Suite 1040
Atlanta GA 30338

National Medical Enterprises Inc.
11620 Wilshire Boulevard
Los Angeles CA 90025

Qualicare
PO Box 24189
New Orleans LA 70184

St Mary's Hospital
1800 E. Lakeside Dr
Decatur IL 62525

The Woodward Group
35 E. Wacker Dr.
Suite 3400
Chicago IL 60601

X-Ray and screening services

Bennett X-Ray Corporation
54 Railroad Avenue
Copiagne NY 11726
Telephone: (516) 691 6100

California X-Ray Co.
2206 W. 7th Street
Los Angeles CA 90057

Du Pont Company X-Ray Products
1007 Market Street
Wilmington DE 19898

Transworld X-Ray Corporation
10210 Pineville Road
Charlotte NC 28210
Telephone: (704) 554 8390

Emergency medical recruitment services

Emergency Consultants Inc.
2240 S. Airport Rd
Traverse City MI 49684

Emergency Medical Services Association
8200 N. Sunrise Boulevard
Plantation FL 33322

Locum Tenens Group Inc.
2301 Bellevue Ave 4-W
Los Angeles CA 90026

Medical Center Ltd
PO Box 309
131 New London Turnpike
Glastonbury CT 06033

National Emergency Services Inc.
PO Box 156
Tiburon CA 94920

National Emergency Services Inc.
4419 Cowan Rd
Tucker GA 30084

National Emergency Services Inc.
9953 Lewis & Clark
St Louis MO 63136

National Emergency Services Inc.
1 Hollow Lane
Lake Success NY 11042

National Emergency Services Inc.
1955 S. Reynolds
Toledo OH 43614

National Emergency Services Inc.
3301 Airport Freeway
Bedford TX 76021

NEEMA Emergency Medical
399 Market St
Suite 400
Philadelphia PA 19106

Pharmaceutical Industry Placement Service
19 Berkeley Pl
Montclair NJ 07042

Spectrum Emergency Care Inc.
970 Executive Pkwy
St Louis MO 63141

Main banks

American National Bank & Trust Company
of Chicago
Bank of America
Chase Manhattan Bank NA
Citibank NA
First National Bank of America

Useful sources of information

Community care: alcoholism

National Council on Alcoholism
1100 17th Street NW
Suite 710
Washington DC 20036
Telephone: (202) 223 1998

733 Third Avenue
New York NY 10017
Telephone: (202) 986 4433

National Council on Drug Abuse
571 West Jackson
Chicago ILL 60606
Telephone: (312) 663 9224

Community care: ambulance service

American Ambulance Association
c/o The David Epstein Group PC
1000 Potomac St NW
Washington DC 2007
Telephone: (202) 337 7360

Community care: general

Asthma & Allergy Foundation of America
1302 18th Street NW
Suite 303
Washington DC 20036
Telephone: (202) 293 2950

Action on Smoking & Health
2013 H Street NW
Washington DC 20006
Telephone: (202) 659 4310

Alexander Graham Bell Association for the
Deaf
3417 Volta Place NW
Washington DC 20007
Telephone: (202) 337 5220

American Diabetes Association
1156 15th Street NW
Suite 302
Washington DC 20005
Telephone: (202) 659 2900

American Foundation for the Blind
1660 L Street NW
Suite 214
Washington DC 20036
Telephone: (202) 467 5997

American Heart Association
1110 Vermont Avenue NW
Suite 820
Washington DC 20036
Telephone: (202) 822 9380

American Cancer Society
1575 I Street NW
Suite 1025
Washington DC 20005
Telephone: (202) 289 0833

American Council of the Blind
1211 Connecticut Avenue NW
Suite 506
Washington DC 20036
Telephone: (202) 833 1251

American Dance Therapy Association
2000 Century Plaza
Suite 108
Columbia
Maryland 21044
Telephone: (301) 997 4040

American Kidney Fund
7315 Wisconsin Avenue
Suite 203E
Bethesda
Maryland 20814
Telephone: (301) 986 1444

American Lung Association
1101 Vermont Avenue NW
Suite 402
Washington DC 20005
Telephone: (202) 289 5057

American National Red Cross
Office of Public Information
17th & D Street NW
Washington DC 20006
Telephone: (202) 737 8300

Arthritis Foundation
1915 I Street NW
Suite 500
Washington DC 20007
Telephone: (202) 543 1810

Cooley's Anemia Foundation
c/o Science & Health Communications
Group Inc
10,000 Falls Road
Suite 306
Potomac
Maryland 20854
Telephone: (301) 983 9773

Cystic Fibrosis Foundation
6000 Executive Boulevard
Suite 510
Rockville
Maryland 20852
Telephone: (301) 881 9130

Endocrine Society
9650 Rockville Pike
Bethesda
Maryland 20814
Telephone: (301) 530 9660

Epilepsy Foundation of America
4351 Garden City Drive
Suite 406
Landover
Maryland 20785
Telephone: (301) 459 3700

Eye Bank Association of America
6560 Fannin
Level 9
Houston, Texas 77030
Telephone: (713) 799 6126

Huntington's Disease Foundation of
America
250 West 57th Street
Suite 2016
New York NY 10107
Telephone: (212) 757 0443

Leukemia Society of America
1625 I Street NW
Suite 923
Washington DC 20006
Telephone: (202) 223 2656

Muscular Dystrophy Association
1800 Massachusetts Avenue NW
Suite 100
Washington DC 20036
Telephone: (202) 466 6450

National Association for Home Care
519 C Street NE
Washington DC 20002
Telephone: (202) 547 7424

National Association for Music Therapy
1133 15th St NW
Washington DC 20005
Telephone: (202) 429 9440

National Association for the Deaf
814 Thayer Ave
Silver Spring
Maryland 20910
Telephone: (301) 587 1788

National Foundation for Cancer Research
7315 Wisconsin Ave
Suite 322W
Bethesda
Maryland 20814
Telephone: (301) 654 1250

National Hemophilia Foundation
c/o Grupenhoff & Endicott
10,000 Falls Rd
Suite 306
Potomac
Maryland 20854
Telephone: (301) 983 9773

National Hospice Organization
1901 North Fort Myer Drive
Suite 402
Arlington
Virginia 22209
Telephone: (703) 243 5900

National Initiative for Glaucoma Control
1140 Connecticut Ave NW
Suite 606
Washington DC 20036
Telephone: (202) 466 4555

National Kidney Foundation
1319 18th Street NW
3rd Floor
Washington DC 20036
Telephone: (202) 659 1373

National Multiple Sclerosis Society
c/o Carley Capital Group
2623 Connecticut Ave NW
Washington DC 20008
Telephone: (202) 328 3272

National Society for Children & Adults with
Autism
1234 Massachusetts Ave NW
Washington DC 20005
Telephone: (202) 783 0125

National Society to Prevent Blindness
79 Madison Ave NY
New York 10016
Telephone: (202) 684 3505

National Spinal Cord Injury Association
2550 M Street NW
Suite 280
Washington DC 20036
Telephone: (202) 293 0202

United Cerebral Palsy Association
425 I Street
Suite 141
Washington DC 20001
Telephone: (202) 842 1266

Community care: geriatrics

Administration on Ageing
Office of Human Development, Dept of
Health & Human Service
Washington DC 20201
Telephone: (202) 245 0724

American Association of Homes for the
Ageing
1050 17th St NW
Suite 779
Washington DC 20036
Telephone: (202) 296 5960

American Association of Retired Persons
1909 K St Northwest
Washington DC 20049
Telephone: (202) 872 4700

National Council on the Ageing
600 Maryland Ave SW
West Wing 100
Washington DC 20024
Telephone: (202) 479 1200

National Council of Senior Citizens
925 15th St NW
Washington DC 20005
Telephone: (202) 347 8800

United States Dept of Health & Human
Service
Administration on Ageing
330 Independence Ave Southwest
Washington DC 20010
Telephone: (202) 245 0188

Solicitors

American Bar Association
1155 East 60th St
Chicago ILL 60637
Telephone: (312) 947 4000

*Business organisations: medical office building
consultants*

Architectural Services
American Institute of Architects
1735 New York Ave NW
Washington DC 20006

Ellerbe, Inc.
1 Appletree Sq.
Bloomington MN 55420

Harold J. Westin and Associates, Inc.
45 E. Eighth St
St Paul MN 55101

Marshall Erdman and Associates, Inc.
51117 University Ave
Madison W1 55705

Medical Construction Management Corp.
5201 Old Middleton Rd
Madison W1 53705

Nationwide Medical-Dental Bidg Corp.
797 Market St
Oregon W1 53575

Professional Office Bidg Inc.
Doctors Park
Madison W1 53705

Business organisations: medical printers

Medical Arts Press
3440 Winnetka Ave
North Minneapolis MN 55427

Physicians' Board Co.
3000 S. Ridgeland Ave
Berwyn IL 60402

*Business organisations: dictation and
transcription equipment*

Dictaphone Corp.
120 Old Post Rd
Rye NY 10580
Telephone: 914-967-6211

IBM Corp.
Parson's Pond Dr.
Franklin Lakes NJ 07417
Telephone: 201-848-1900

Lanier Business Products
1700 Chantilly Dr. NE
Atlanta GA 30324
Telephone: 404-329-8000

Norelco Corp.
Phillips Business Systems, Inc.
810 Woodbury Rd
Woodbury NY 11797
Telephone: 516-921-9310

Sanyo Business Systems Corp.
51 Joseph St
Moonachie NJ 07074
Telephone: 201-440-9300

Sony Corp. of America
9 W. Fifty-seventh St
New York NY 10019
Telephone: 212-371-5800

Business organisations: filing equipment

Business Systems & Security Marketing
Association, Inc.
835 S. 130th St
Omaha NE 68154
Telephone: 402-333-6780

Kardex Systems, Inc.
PO Box 171
Marietta
Ohio 45750
Telephone: 800-848-9761

Lundia Myers Industries, Inc.
600 Capitol Way
Jacksonville IL 62650
Telephone: 217-243-8585

Steelcase Corp.
1120 Thirty-sixth St
Grand Rapids MI 49508
Telephone: 616-274-2710

Supreme Equipment & Systems Corp.
170 Fifty-third St
Brooklyn NY 11232
Telephone: 212-492-7777

Tab Products Corp.
269 Hanover
Palo Alto CA 94300
Telephone: 415-493-5790

White Power Files, Inc.
850 Springfield Rd
Union NJ 07083
Telephone: 201-687-9522

Fire equipment

Arson Resource Center
Office of Planning & Education
US Fire Administration
Washington DC 20472
Telephone: (202) 254 7840

National Fire Protection Association
Battery March Park
Quincy MA 02269
Telephone: (617) 328 9290

National Burglar & Fire Alarms Association
1101 Connecticut Ave
Washington DC 20036
Telephone: (202) 857 1130

Motoring organisations

Automobile Insurance Plans Service Office
733 Third Ave
New York NY 10017
Telephone: (212) 867 0500

Index

Accountant, 33
  advice, 32–3
  finding, 34
  requirement, 33
  responsibilities, 33, 63
Account forms, 102–3
Accounts, 54–60
  bank, 58
  books, required, 57–9
  collection, 122–127
  keeping, 56
  overdue, 124–6
  profit and loss, 44
  wages and salaries, 59–60, 133–4
Acts of Parliament, 154
Advertising, 76–9
  local press, 78
  telephone directories, 78–9
  writing letters, 77
  for staff, 129–130
  yellow pages, 96
Advice, professional, 32–36
  architect, 22
  accountant, 33
  bank, 35–6, 50–1
  solicitor, 33–4, 85
  stockbroker, 64
Agency staff, 137–8
Allowances, 62–3
Analysis ledger, 56–8
Ansaphone, 94
Answering services, 94–5
Appointments
  book, 76, 103
  cards, 102, 122
  hospital patients, 146
  reminders, 122
  scheduling, 120–2, 141
Assets, 46–7
  current, 46–7
  fixed, 46–7
  purchasing a practice, 28–30
  tangible, 39–40
Assistant, 15
Associate practice, 14

Australia, 157–166
  government organisations, 157
  medical insurance, 161–4
  private hospitals, 164–5
  professional organisations, 157–161
  useful sources of information, 165

Balance sheet, 46–7
Bank
  accounts and statements, 58–9
  approaching the bank, 50–1
  loan, 52
  manager, 35–6
  references and information, 51
  overdrafts, 52
  savings and building societies, 50, 53
Belgium, 167–9
  government organisations, 167
  professional organisations, 167–9
  useful sources of information, 169
Books
  accounts, 57–9
  address, 103–4
  analysis, 56–8
  appointment, 103
  cash, 56–8
  day, 58
  petty cash, 59
  reference, 105
Break even chart, 48–9
Budgeting, 44–50

Call systems, 95
Canada, 170–177
  government organisations, 170–1
  medical insurance, 175–7
  private hospitals, 177
  professional organisations, 171–5
  useful sources of information, 177
Capital, 37–8
  allowances, 62–3
  initial, 38

partnership, 13
working, 38
Car, 11, 105–6
insurance, 82
telephone and cellular network, 95–6
Cash
book, 56–8
deposits, 59
flow, 44–5
insurance 83–4
petty, 59
Chaperones, 73–4
Communications, 93–6
Companies
limited, 14, 87
pharmaceutical and manufacturing, 119–120
Complaints, 75–76
Computers, 98–101
advantages and disadvantages, 100
Data Protection Act, 100–1
Conduct, professional, 74–6
complaints from a patient, 75–6
disciplinary procedures, 74–5
rules of, 66, 74
Confidentiality, 70–2
Consent, 69–70
adults, 69–70
informed, 70, 144
minors, 70
Consultancy, hospital, 138–9
Consultations, 116–118
Consulting room, 115–118
Contracts
hospital practitioner, 141–144
insurance, 80
landlord, 26
patient, 67–8
staff, 60, 133–4
Conveyancing, 87
Costs
advisers, 34
budgeting and forecasting, 44–50
hidden, 40–1
running, 40
starting, 39
tax allowable costs, 62–3
Credit cards, 123–4
Credit control, 124–126

Day book, 58
Debt collection, 29
commercial agency, 124–5
courts, 125

credit control, 124–6
solicitor's letter, 124
Decor, 108–111
Delegation, 128–9
Denmark, 178–9
government organisations, 178
medical insurance, 179
professional organisations, 178
Deposits, 59
Depreciation, 54, 63
Disciplinary procedures, 74–5
Discharging patients, 118, 145
Domiciliary practice, 11–12, 145
Doorplate, 110–111
Drugs, 74, 83, 145

Eire, 180–182
government organisations, 180
medical insurance, 181
private hospitals, 181
professional organisations 180–1
useful sources of information, 182
Emergency
staff, 137–8
telephone calls, 114
Employer
legal liabilities, 72–3
Liability Act, 134, 137
liability insurance, 82
relationships with employees 134–5
Equipment, 92–3, 115–6, 119–120
buying, 119–120
consulting room, 115–116
hospital, 144
office, 92–3
purchasing assets and stock, 29
service engineer, 120
Estate agent, 20–1, 87
Estimates, 22
Ethics, 66
Expenses, 62–3
Experience, 3–4

Fees
account forms, 102–3
book (day book), 58
complaints, 75
costing, 41–2
credit control, 124–6
death of a patient, 126
debt collection, 124–5
hospital, 146
income, 6, 7–8
income chart, 48–9

reminders, 65
tracing a patient, 125–6
treatment of another practitioner, 118
Filing equipment, 96–7
Filing systems, 97–101
Finance, 37–65
    long term planning, 38–9
    purchasing a practice, 28–32
    short-term planning, 38
    sources of, 50–4
Finance and leasing companies, 53–4
Fire precautions, 24–5
    extinguishers, 91
Fixtures and fittings
    office, 89–97
    purchasing, 29–30
Forecasting and budgeting, 46–50
Freehold premises, 10, 25–6

Goodwill, 30–1
Government grants, 53
Group practice, 14

Health, 5–7
History of private practice, 148–9
Holidays, 4, 5, 143
    staff, 134
Home practice, 9–10, 25–6, 62–3
Hong Kong, 183–4
    government organisations, 183
    medical insurance, 183
    private hospitals, 184
    professional organisations, 183
    useful sources of information, 184
Hospital practice management, 139–147
    admitting rights, 141
    discharging patients, 145–6
    fees, 146
    follow-up appointments, 146
    informed consent, 144–5
    record keeping, 145–6
    scheduling visits, 141

Income, 6, 7–8
    financial planning and management, 36–65
Injections, 74
Inland revenue, 60–4
Insurance, 9, 79–84
    broker, 34–5
    car, 82

contract, 80
drugs, 83
legal liability, 81–2
life policies, 84
    pensions, 64, 84
medical practice and premises, 80–2
money, 83–4
mortgage, 84
national insurance contributions, 60–1
permanent health, 83
personnel accident, 82–3
professional, 81
private medical, 83, 150
public liability, 81–2
Interviews
    hospital practice, 142
    of staff, 130–2
Investment advice, 64
Ireland, Northern 215
Irish Republic, 180–182

Japan, 185
Job description, 129, 142

Landlord and Tenant Act, 26
Law, 66–74
    Acts of Parliament, 154
    advertising, 76–9
    confidentiality, 70–2
    consent, 69–70, 144
    contract with the patient, 67–8
    courts, 85, 125
    debtors, 124–5
    negligence, 67–9
    patient damages, 68
    standards of care, 69
    vicarious liability, 72–4
Leasehold property, 10, 26
Leasing companies, 53–4
Legacies, patients, 88
Letterheads, 101
Liabilities, 46–7
Licences, 24
Limited company, 14, 87
Liquidity, 44
Loans, 50–4
Local authorities, 22–24
Locum, 15, 73, 137
Loss account, profit and, 44

Marriage and tax, 61–2
Medical facilities, local, 19–20

Mortgage insurance, 84

Name of practice, 77
National Health Service
    founding, 149
    and private practice, 1, 140, 151
National Insurance, 60–1
    Act (1911), 149
Needs
    personal, 2–3, 18–9, 41
    financial, 36–65
    income, 6, 7–8
Negligence, 67–9
Netherlands, 186–188
    government organisations, 186
    medical insurance, 187–8
    professional organisations, 186–7
New Zealand, 189–190
    government organisations, 189
    medical insurance, 189
    professional organisations, 189
    useful sources of information, 190
Northern Ireland, 215
Norway, 191

Office, planning and management,
    89–107
    business equipment, 92–3
    communications, 93–6
    filing equipment and systems
        96–101
    furniture, 89–90
    printing and stationery, 101–4
    professional cards, 101
    professional letterheads, 101

Partnership, 13–14, 52, 85
    advantages, 13
    agreements, 13, 85–6
    car ownership, 106
    duration, 86
    partnership capital, 52
    salaried partners, 52
    sleeping partner, 52
Part-time practice, 14–5
Patients
    appointments, 120–2, 141
    consultations, 116–118
    complaints, 75–6
    consent, 69–70, 141
    discharging, 118, 145
    hospital, 139–147
    legacies, 88

other professionals, 118
    records, 76, 97–101
    reminders, 122
    time factor, 4, 5, 143
Pay as you earn, PAYE, 60
Pensions, 64, 144
Personnel, 128–138
Petty cash book, 59
Planning
    long-term, 38
    premises, 108–127
    permission, 23–4
    short-term, 38
    size and layout, 21–2
Police, 87
Practice, private
    choosing where, 17–20
    community need, 17, 150
    location, 17–20
    – NHS interaction, 140, 151
    policies, 134–5
    purchasing, 27–32
    selling, 87
    starting, 17–36
    ways to practise, 12–15
        association, 14
        assistant, 15
        limited company, 14, 87
        partnership, 13–14, 52, 85
        single-handed, 12–13
Practitioner
    demands on, 1–3
    ethics, 66
    experience and training, 3–4
    health, 5–7
    insurance, 9, 79–84
    legal implications, 66–79
    needs, 18–19
    other health professionals, 8, 9
    personal appearance, 5, 116
    personality, 3
    professional conduct, 74–6
    professional organisation, 8
    time factor, 4, 5, 11, 22–3, 143
    training, 4
Premises, 10–11, 28–9
    acquiring, 20–32
    conveyancing, 87
    freehold, 10, 25–6
    leasehold, 10, 26
    location, 17–20
    purchasing, 27–32
    renting, 10–11, 26–7
    size and layout, 21–2
    viewing and choosing, 24–5
Printing, 101–104

appointment cards, 102
letterheads, 101
logo, 101
medical record cards, 103
professional cards, 101, 102
Professional advisers, 32–36
Profit and loss account, 44
Publicity and the media, 78–9
Purchasing a practice, 27–32
evaluating the assets, 28–31
negotiation, 31

Quotations, 22

Receptionist, 113–115
Reception room, 111–113
call systems, 95
decor, 108–111
furnishings, 112–113
notices, 115
Records
cards, 103
hospital, 145
legal requirements, 76, 97–101
medical, 4, 76, 103
purchasing, 30
Recruitment agencies, 137–8
Reference books, 105
Relationships
approaching other practitioners, 8–9
patients, 116
staff, 132, 135–7
treating other professionals, 118
Renting, 10–11, 26–7
Retirement and pensions, 64

Safe, 90
Safety precautions, 40, 134
fire precautions, 24–5
Salaries, 53, 59–60, 133–4
salaried partners, 53
staff, 59–60, 133–4
Sale of goods, 78, 119–120
Savings, 50
Scheduling, 120
hospital patients, 141
Secretary, 113–115
Security, 9, 24, 90
Selling a practice, 87
evaluation of assets, 29–31
goodwill, 30–1
Service engineer, 120
Sick leave

hospital practitioner, 143
staff, 134
Single handed practice, 12–13
Solicitor, 33–4, 85–88
Solo practice, 12–13
South Africa, 192
Staff employment, 128–138
additional costing, 48–9
contracts, 60, 133–4
delegation of responsibility, 128–9
discharging, 137
emergency, 137–8
interviews, 130–2
keeping, 132
management and training, 135–6
practice policies, 134–5
promotion, 136
purchasing a practice, 31
recruitment and advertising, 129–130
references, 133–4
relatives, 132
selection, 132
Staff room, 90
Statements
bank, 58–9
income and expenditure, 43
Stress, 6–7
Sweden, 194
Switzerland, 195

Taxation, 60–4
allowable expenses, 62–3
and marriage, 61–2
pay as you earn PAYE, 60
provision of payment, 41
tax year, 61
value added tax VAT, 63
Telephone and calling services, 93–6
call divertors, 95
car, 95–6
cellular network, 96
directories, 78, 79, 96
reminders, 122
yellow pages, 78, 79, 96
Theft
insurance, 83–4
prevention, 90
Time
hospital visits, 143
management, 4–5
premises and estimates, 22–3
travelling, 11
Title of practice, 77
Training
practitioner, 3–4

staff, 135–6

United Kingdom, 196–214
    government organisations, 196
    medical insurance, 198–9
    Northern Ireland, 215
    private hospitals, 199–206
    professional organisations, 196–8
    useful sources of information,
        207–14
United States of America, 216–31
    government organisations, 216–9
    medical insurance, 220–26
    private hospitals, 226–8
    professional organisations, 219–20
    useful sources of information,
        228–31

Value Added Tax, 63
Vendor, 30–1
    conveyancing, 87
    evaluation of assets, 28–31
    goodwill, 30–1
Visiting hospitals, 141

Wages and salaries, 59–60, 133–4
Waiting room, 111–113
Wife, taxation, 61–2
Will, 88
Word processor, 92

Yellow pages, 78, 79, 96